Medicine Outside Four Walls

Editors

KIM ZUBER
JANE S. DAVIS

PHYSICIAN ASSISTANT CLINICS

www.physicianassistant.theclinics.com

Consulting Editors
KIM ZUBER
JANE S. DAVIS

April 2024 • Volume 9 • Number 2

ELSEVIER

1600 John F. Kennedy Boulevard • Suite 1800 • Philadelphia, Pennsylvania, 19103-2899

http://www.theclinics.com

PHYSICIAN ASSISTANT CLINICS Volume 9, Number 2
April 2024 ISSN 2405-7991, ISBN-13: 978-0-443-18348-5

Editor: Taylor Hayes
Developmental Editor: Saswoti Nath

Physician Assistant Clinics (ISSN: 2405–7991) is published quarterly by Elsevier Inc., 360 Park Avenue South, New York, NY 10010-1710. Months of issue are January, April, July, and October. Periodicals postage paid at New York, NY and additional mailing offices. Subscription prices are $155.00 per year (US individuals), $100.00 (US students), $150.00 (Canadian individuals), $100.00 (Canadian students), $150.00 (international individuals), and $100.00 (international students). For institutional access pricing please contact Customer Service via the contact information below. Foreign air speed delivery is included in all *Clinics* subscription prices. All prices are subject to change without notice. POSTMASTER: Send address changes to *Physician Assistant Clinics*, Elsevier Periodicals Customer Service, 11830 Westline Industrial Drive, St. Louis, MO 63146. Customer Service Health Sciences Division, Subscription Customer Service, 3251 Riverport Lane, Maryland Heights, MO 63043. **Customer Service: 1-800-654-2452 (U.S. and Canada); 314-447-8871 (outside U.S. and Canada). Fax: 314-447-8029. E-mail: journalscustomerservice-usa@elsevier.com (for print support); journalsonlinesupport-usa@elsevier.com (for online support).**

Reprints. For copies of 100 or more, of articles in this publication, please contact the Commercial Reprints Department, Elsevier Inc., 360 Park Avenue South, New York, NY 10010-1710. Tel. 212-633-3874; Fax: 212-633-3820; E-mail: reprints@elsevier.com.

Physician Assistant Clinics is covered in *EMBASE/Excerpta Medica and ESCI*.

PROGRAM OBJECTIVE
The goal of the *Physician Assistant Clinics* is to keep practicing physician assistants up to date with current clinical practice by providing timely articles reviewing the state of the art in patient care.

TARGET AUDIENCE
Physician Assistants and other healthcare professionals

LEARNING OBJECTIVES
Upon completion of this activity, participants will be able to:
1. Review methods that positively contribute to health education efficacy and equity.
2. Discuss modalities that help deliver quality and cost-effective healthcare to highly vulnerable populations.
3. Recognize wilderness medicine has moved to an evidence-based professional specialty and may be practiced by any clinician who assists in natural disasters.

ACCREDITATION
The Elsevier Office of Continuing Medical Education (EOCME) is accredited by the Accreditation Council for Continuing Medical Education (ACCME) to provide continuing medical education for physicians.

The EOCME designates this journal-based CME activity for a maximum of 16 *AMA PRA Category 1 Credit*(s)™. Physicians should claim only the credit commensurate with the extent of their participation in the activity.

All other health care professionals requesting continuing education credit for this enduring material will be issued a certificate of participation.

DISCLOSURE OF CONFLICTS OF INTEREST
The EOCME assesses conflict of interest with its instructors, faculty, planners, and other individuals who are in a position to control the content of CME activities. All relevant conflicts of interest that are identified are thoroughly vetted by EOCME for fair balance, scientific objectivity, and patient care recommendations. EOCME is committed to providing its learners with CME activities that promote improvements or quality in healthcare and not a specific proprietary business or a commercial interest.

The planning committee, staff, authors, and editors listed below have identified no financial relationships or relationships to products or devices they or their spouse/life partner have with commercial interest related to the content of this CME activity:
Caitlin Arnone, MPAS, PA-C, CRA; Alexander J. Axtell, MPAS, PA-C, FAWM; Audra Baca, MPH, CHES; Keri Baker, MS, MSN, ENP, FNP-C; Brandon R. Beattie, MMSc, PA-C; J. Pearce Beissinger, MS, PA-C, DiMM; Janelle Bludorn, MS, PA-C; Mirela Bruza-Augatis, MS, PA-C; Jane S. Davis, DNP; Fatima Elgarguri, BS, PA/MPH-S; Darcie Evans; Jessica Gehner, MD; Seth C. Hawkins, MD, W/NR-EMT; Rodney Ho, PhD, MPAS, MPH, PA-C, Psychiatry-CAQ; Kerri Jack, MHS, PA-C; Jenny Jordan, RN, BSN; Alan M. Keating, MPAS, PA-C; Kothainayaki Kulanthaivelu, BCA, MBA; Stephanie Lareau, MD; Linda Laskowski-Jones, MS, APRN, ACNS-BC, CEN, NEA-BC, FAWM; Michelle Littlejohn; John S. Lynch, DMSc, PA-C, DFAAPA; Anna Mardis; Rebecca Maxson, PharmD, BCPS; Joshua Nichols, MD; Eric Olsen, PA-C; Mary Showstark, MPAS, PA-C; Derrick Varner, PhD, PA-C, DFAAPA, RDMS; Kim Zuber, PA-C

UNAPPROVED/OFF-LABEL USE DISCLOSURE
The EOCME requires CME faculty to disclose to the participants:
1. When products or procedures being discussed are off-label, unlabelled, experimental, and/or investigational (not US Food and Drug Administration [FDA] approved); and
2. Any limitations on the information presented, such as data that are preliminary or that represent ongoing research, interim analyses, and/or unsupported opinions. Faculty may discuss information about pharmaceutical agents that is outside of FDA-approved labelling. This information is intended solely for CME and is not intended to promote off-label use of these medications. If you have any questions, contact the medical affairs department of the manufacturer for the most recent prescribing information.

TO ENROLL
The CME program is available to all *Physician Assistant Clinics* subscribers at no additional fee. To subscribe to the *Physician Assistant Clinics*, call customer service at 1-800-654-2452 or sign up online at www.physicianassistant.theclinics.com.

METHOD OF PARTICIPATION

In order to claim credit, participants must complete the following:

1. Complete enrolment as indicated above
2. Read the activity
3. Complete the CME Test and Evaluation. Participants must achieve a score of 70% on the test. All CME Tests and Evaluations must be completed online

CME INQUIRIES/SPECIAL NEEDS

For all CME inquiries or special needs, please contact elsevierCME@elsevier.com.

Contributors

CONSULTING EDITORS

KIM ZUBER, PA-C
Executive Director, American Academy of Nephrology PAs, Melbourne, Florida, USA

JANE S. DAVIS, DNP
Nurse Practitioner, Division of Nephrology, University of Alabama at Birmingham, Birmingham, Alabama, USA

EDITORS

KIM ZUBER, PA-C
Executive Director, American Academy of Nephrology PAs, Melbourne, Florida, USA

JANE S. DAVIS, DNP
Nurse Practitioner, Division of Nephrology, University of Alabama at Birmingham, Birmingham, Alabama, USA

AUTHORS

CAITLIN ARNONE, MPAS, PA-C, CRA
Associate Medical Safety Officer, Thermo Fisher Scientific, Wilmington, North Carolina, USA

ALEXANDER J. AXTELL, MPAS, PA-C, FAWM
Physician Assistant, Emergency Medicine, Carilion Clinic, Virginia Tech Carilion, Roanoke, Virginia, USA

AUDRA BACA, MPH, CHES
Master of Global Health and Medical Anthropology (in process), CHES, Oregon City, Oregon, USA

KERI BAKER, MS, MSN, ENP, FNP-C
Family and Emergency Medicine Nurse Practitioner, Roanoke, Virginia, USA

BRANDON R. BEATTIE, MMSc, PA-C
Assistant Professor, Director of Didactic Education, The George Washington University, Department of PA Studies, School of Medicine and Health Sciences, Washington, DC, USA

JASON PEARCE BEISSINGER, MS, PA-C, DiMM
Captain, ORANG, 142d MDG Det-1, 102d Oregon CBRNE-CERFP, Assistant Medical Director, Portland Mountain Rescue, Happy Valley, Oregan, USA

JANELLE BLUDORN, MS, PA-C
Assistant Professor, Department of Family Medicine and Community Health, Duke University School of Medicine, Durham, North Carolina, USA

MIRELA BRUZA-AUGATIS, MS, PA-C
Research Scientist, Exams and Research, Assistant Professor, Seton Hall University, National Commission on Certification of Physician Assistants, Johns Creek, Georgia, USA

JANE S. DAVIS, DNP
Nurse Practitioner, Division of Nephrology, University of Alabama at Birmingham, Birmingham, Alabama, USA

FATIMA ELGARGURI, BS, PA/MPH-S
Department of PA Studies, The George Washington University, School of Medicine and Health Sciences, Washington, DC, USA

DARCIE EVANS, PharmD
Candidate 2024, Auburn University Harrison College of Pharmacy, Auburn, Alabama, USA

JESSICA GEHNER, MD
Emergency Medicine Physician, Department of Emergency Medicine, Wilderness Medicine Fellowship Assistant Director, Virginia Tech Carilion, Roanoke, Virginia, USA

SETH C. HAWKINS, MD, W/NR-EMT
Associate Professor, Department of Emergency Medicine, Wake Forest University, Associate Director, Wake Forest Wilderness Medicine Fellowship, Affiliate Faculty, Department of Anthropology, Wake Forest, Winston-Salem, North Carolina, USA; Medical Director, NC Department of Natural and Cultural Resources (State Parks), Raleigh, North Carolina, USA

RODNEY HO, PhD, MPAS, MPH, PA-C
Psychiatry-CAQ, Rocky Mountain University, Provo, Utah, USA

KERRI JACK, MHS, PA-C
Assistant Professor, Clinical Coordinator, Chatham University Master of PA Studies Program, Pittsburgh, Pennsylvania, USA

JENNY JORDAN, RN, BSN
Executive Director, Sacred Valley Health, Pilochuasi s/n, Ollantaytambo, Cusco, Peru

ALAN M. KEATING, MPAS, PA-C
Physician Assistant, University of Nebraska Medical Center, Snellville, Georgia, USA

STEPHANIE LAREAU, MD
Associate Professor, Department of Emergency Medicine, Carilion Clinic, Virginia Tech Carilion School of Medicine, Roanoke, Virginia, USA

LINDA LASKOWSKI-JONES, MS, APRN, ACNS-BC, CEN, NEA-BC, FAWM
Executive Director, Appalachian Center for Wilderness Medicine, Morganton, North Carolina, USA; Blue Mountain Ski Patrol, Palmerton, Pennsylvania, USA; Editor-in-Chief: *Nursing2024*, Wolters Kluwer, Philadelphia, Pennsylvania, USA

JOHN S. LYNCH, DMSc, PA-C, DFAAPA
Physician Assistant, Tidewater Physician Multispecialty Group, Gastroenterology Williamsburg, Williamsburg, Virginia, USA

ANNA MARDIS, PharmD
Candidate 2024, Auburn University Harrison College of Pharmacy, Auburn, Alabama, USA

REBECCA MAXSON, PharmD, BCPS
Associate Clinical Professor, Auburn University Harrison College of Pharmacy, Auburn, Alabama, USA

JOSHUA NICHOLS, MD
Clinical Preceptor, Emergency Medicine Physician, Virginia Tech Carilion School of Medicine, Roanoke, Virginia, USA

ERIC OLSEN, PA-C
Physician Assistant, Department of Emergency Medicine, Carilion Clinic, Roanoke, Virginia, USA

MARY SHOWSTARK, MPAS, PA-C
Assistant Professor Adjunct, Affiliate Faculty, Yale Institute for Global Health Instructor, Yale School of Medicine Physician Assistant Online Program, Yale University, New Haven, Connecticut, USA

DERRICK VARNER, PhD, PA-C, DFAAPA, RDMS
Chatham University Master of PA Studies Program, Woodland Road, Pittsburgh, Pennsylvania, USA

KIM ZUBER, PA-C
Executive Director, American Academy of Nephrology PAs, Melbourne, Florida, USA

Contents

As medical providers, our families and friends often come to us for advice or evaluation, even on topics outside of our scope of practice. In emergencies, we are often called on to treat the injured or ill. We accept this responsibility in non-office settings because we know the hospital is nearby. However, in the wilderness, it is a different situation. Our treatment of the injured and ill has the added dynamics of limited supplies and the distance to advanced care. This article explores the basic principles of wilderness medicine triage and treatment principles needed to render care in challenging surroundings.

Many medical advances have stemmed from the casualties of war and have changed civilian medicine in concrete ways. Each military service is responsible for a specific part of the environment: sea, land, air, and space. Navy medics are experts in cold water injury exposures and deep-sea explorations. Through their care of the Marines, they have developed multilevel trauma interventions and triage. The Army is responsible for land-based medical care leading to advancements in treating and stabilizing life-threatening injuries in harsh environments.

Originally coined in 1992, the term street medicine describes an expanding modality providing high-quality, cost-effective healthcare to vulnerable populations who may not otherwise engage in routine healthcare, especially those experiencing homelessness. Care rendered includes primary care services, basic wound care, urgent care needs, and mental healthcare. Mobile medicine practitioners deliver similar care as their street medicine colleagues but may also provide mammography and ophthalmology screening. While street medicine practitioners carry all of their equipment with them, mobile medicine practitioners benefit from having more equipment and resources at their disposal from the mobile health clinics.

Valley Health in rural Peru has solved this issue by the development of a local community health worker program. By training and using local women to manage and run the program, cultural, geographic, and social practices are maintained for a sustainable health promotion program. The Sacred Valley Health outreach in partnership with indigenous, high-altitude communities in the Peruvian Andes can be replicated in other areas with austere medical circumstances.

The golden age of wilderness medicine began in the 1970s with the introduction of formal classes and certifications. As wilderness medicine moves in the twenty-first century, more standardization, consensus, increased professionalism and career pathways, and evidence-based practices are the hallmark modern wilderness medicine. Wilderness Emergency Medical Services (EMS), the formal and preplanned delivery of wilderness medicine by health care professionals, can include search and rescue teams, ski patrols, rangers, mountain rescue teams, the military, and natural disaster teams. These are all fertile areas in which health care practitioners can contribute critical skills and play important roles.

Wilderness medicine fellowships are an exciting opportunity for physicians, PAs and NPs. Although there are a limited number of fellowship programs, they offer unique opportunities for those interested in practicing outside traditional settings combined with a love for the outdoors. Wilderness medicine has a formal fellowship track and has recently changed to a match system. Fellowships are found in multiple states across the country and are 1 year in duration. Physician applicants must be postfellowship, and 2 of the programs accept PAs and NPs. PA/NP applications require a minimum of 2 years in practice before being eligible for fellowship.

Considerations and successful strategies in planning and delivering effective wilderness medicine training require forethought and planning. Training topics include developing effective lectures, hands-on experiences with improvised equipment, and the use of realistic scenarios with simulated patients and human actors. The use of moulage and other props promotes realism, stimulates critical thinking, and promotes effective problem solving in an austere or resource-limited environment. Wilderness medicine practice opportunities can be found in a variety of real-world settings, from observation experiences to hands-on practice in immersion programs.

Providing medical support for ultra-endurance running events requires organization and a thorough pre-race plan to ensure timely and effective care to the injured runner(s). Medical kits should be designed/assembled to care for conditions likely to be encountered in the specific race setting. In order to build an adequate medical kit, categorize conditions into "serious but uncommon"and "less serious but more common" then outline specific supplies needed for each situation. A preplanned communication structure and race day communication strategies is imperative for maintaining an effective response to race medical emergencies.

Altitude-related illness occurs as a result of inadequate acclimatization. The mainstay of prevention is a slow-graded ascent profile, which gives the body time to respond to a low-oxygen environment. Diagnosis of these conditions is often difficult in resource-limited environments, so history and physical examination are key in identifying patients who will require descent and evacuation. Treatment modalities, supplemental oxygen, portable hyperbaric chambers, and medications are all temporizing measures until the patient can be safely evacuated to a lower elevation.

The roles of the mountain rescuer go beyond the walls of clinic and hospital. Indeed, mountain rescuers may come from all walks of life: healthcare, law, ministry, engineering, military, and even carpentry. Collectively, these teammates bring together their unique blend of skills that, along with medical and technical rescue training, successfully execute a mountain rescue mission. The sacrifice of time for training and missions comes at the cost of personal pursuits. Rescuers are motivated by the greater good of volunteering for the sake of others.

Scuba diving attracts more than 6 million divers worldwide for an average of 30 million dives per week. Three large organizations; the Center for Disease Control and Prevention, the Divers Alert Network, and the Undersea and Hyperbaric Society have developed programs to train practitioners on dive physicals, educate the public on dive safety, and collect data on mortality and morbidity worldwide. We present the most recent medical data available on scuba diving with a discussion of diagnosis of serious adverse events. We discuss both western and eastern style treatments.

Eric Olsen and Stephanie Lareau

Within austere and wilderness environments medical care is often provided by teams made up of many different types of health care providers. Search and rescue (SAR) teams are often composed of lay people with training including wilderness first aid or wilderness first responder and health care professionals including emergency medical technicians , paramedics, registered nurses, nurse practitioners, physician assistants (PAs), and/or physicians. A survey of SAR teams in the Intermountain West States showed 66% of members had first aid/cardiopulmonary resuscitation (CPR) training, 17%–emergency medical responders, 10%—emergency medical technicians, 3%–advanced emergency medical technicians, 2%—paramedics, 1%–registered nurses, 0%—PAs, and 1%—physicians.

PHYSICIAN ASSISTANT CLINICS

FORTHCOMING ISSUES

July 2024
Gender Minority Medicine
Diane Bruessow, *Editor*

October 2024
**Advances in Patient Education: An
Integrated Approach**
Lucy W. Kibe and Gerald Kayingo, *Editors*

January 2025
Neurology
Amy Dix, *Editor*

RECENT ISSUES

January 2024
General Orthopedics
Kara-Ann Valentine, *Editor*

October 2023
Allergy, Asthma, and Immunology
Gabriel Ortiz, *Editor*

July 2023
**Emerging and Re-Emerging Infectious
Disease**
Gerald Kayingo, *Editor*

SERIES OF RELATED INTEREST

Primary Care: Clinics in Office Practice
https://www.primarycare.theclinics.com/
Emergency Medicine Clinics and Medical Clinics
https://www.orthopedic.theclinics.com/

Foreword
Medicine on Your Own

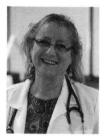 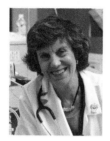

Kim Zuber, PA-C   Jane S. Davis, DNP
Consulting Editors

We've all seen the movie: daring rescue of an injured hiker amid the blizzard of the century. Or there is the plane crash in the remote location and fortunately medical personnel are on board and uninjured. They then deliver first-class medical care under unfavorable conditions. For extra drama, they may even perform surgery with only a flashlight for illumination. And there is always the MASH unit made popular by the long-running TV show.

Medical emergencies are not confined to the emergency department (ED). Many of us have witnessed a car accident, assisted with an orthopedic issue at a kid's sports game, responded to a request for medical help while on a flight, or helped with an issue at a campground, hike, or outdoor event. Even if you have not done so yet, during your career you will. This issue of *Physician Assistant Clinics* is dedicated to you.

It is as natural for us to jump in and assist with medical issues "outside four walls" as it is "inside the four walls" of the facilities where we work and teach. With the assistance of Randy Howell, PA wilderness expert, this issue of *Physician Assistant Clinics* has assembled experts in multiple areas to teach us how to manage patients outside of traditional settings from the depths to the heights. We learn how to treat the dive accident, the high-altitude event, the snow and ski issues, the hypothermia, the running disaster, and many other challenging encounters. In addition to the emergency event, we also get a look at training locals to deliver basic health care and education in remote villages. Because most military medicine is practiced outside four walls, our active-duty colleagues tell us of the ins and outs of their training and the issues faced.

When discussing medicine outside the traditional settings, the term "austere" is often employed. While this may suggest harsh living conditions, in wilderness medicine it is used to describe an environment with limited resources. It can apply equally to a hospital at the base of Mt Everest in Nepal to a MASH unit in an area of conflict to a

Physician Assist Clin 9 (2024) xv–xvi
https://doi.org/10.1016/j.cpha.2023.11.007
2405-7991/24/© 2023 Published by Elsevier Inc.

makeshift clinic in a third-world setting to an elementary school set up as an evacuation center during a fire or hurricane.

Although most of us practice in traditional settings, we do not live in bubbles. Emergencies have no respect for clinic hours, days of the week, or settings. They can and do occur in airplanes, in the grocery store, and while we are relaxing on vacations. This issue highlights many of the sites, complications, and adjustments that can occur when we practice medicine "outside four walls."

Keating takes us on an overview of medicine outside the ER, followed by Ho, Varner, and Beissinger explaining the history and application of military medicine. We don't have to go far to see health care needs; often we see them every day, near our homes or work. Beattie and El-Garguri describe delivering health care to unhoused patients where they are. Arnone, Jack, and Bludorm highlight venomous exposures on land, air, and sea. Mardis, Evans, and Maxson explore the dangers in that attractive plant growing by the trail....or in your yard or home. Lynch highlights the bugs to avoid when traveling or even those who have "moved" into our home territories. The Centers for Disease Control and Prevention (CDC) is warning that what used to be endemic areas is expanding, and thus, bringing a bacterium to us where we live and work.

Showstark and Bruza-Augatis take us beyond the classroom and the United States to tell us about global heath opportunities. An issue with international health care outreach is the lack of consistency and follow-up. Jordan, Baca, and Baker introduce a project in a remote village in Peru that utilizes locals trained to provide basic health care to solve this issue.

Now we move into the "true wilderness" with Hawkins as our guide. He has trained many physicians, PAs, and nurse practitioners (NPs) and highlights the importance of working as a team to handle emergencies outside of four walls. Axell explains the "official" fellowship programs available for PAs and NPs, while Laskowski-Jones guides us through developing wilderness medicine training and how to implement skills learned. Nichols, Olsen, and Lareau describe delivering care during ultramarathons. Gehner takes us to the heights for altitude medicine, and Beissinger describes managing high-altitude emergencies. Sometimes the danger comes from nature itself. Davis and Zuber take us to the ocean depths for a look at dive medicine.

And as important as technical skills are, they are not the only important thing in the wilderness. Olsen and Lareau stress the importance of the interdisciplinary team, especially when you are not near medical facilities. Moving beyond your comfort zone is always challenging, but with insights from these authors, it is possible. And it may provide new opportunities!

Kim Zuber, PA-C
American Academy of Nephrology PAs
Melbourne, FL 32940, USA

Jane S. Davis, DNP
University of Alabama at Birmingham
728 Richard Arrington Boulevard South
Birmingham, AL 35233, USA

E-mail addresses:
zuberkim@yahoo.com (K. Zuber)
jsdavis@uabmc.edu (J.S. Davis)

Wilderness Injuries and Illnesses

When the Emergency Room Is Not "Just Around the Corner"

Alan M. Keating, MPAS, PA-C

KEYWORDS

- Wilderness medicine • Wilderness triage • ABCDEs of wilderness injury assessment
- Injury and illness treatment • Stabilization

KEY POINTS

- Emergent wilderness medicine treatment must be performed quickly and efficiently but with the added difficulty of harsh environments.
- Goals of wilderness medicine are rapid assessment, stabilization, treatment, protection from the environment, and preparation for evacuation.
- A proper evaluation of acute injuries and illnesses will achieve these goals and give the patient the needed time for survival.
- Modern triage principles are necessary for immediate patient assessment in the wilderness.

INTRODUCTION

The practice of medicine usually occurs in a quiet, clean, and often sterile environment. Patients wait for the provider in the room with most of the supplies at hand. Everything is in order, and everything is in its place. Now, let's step out of those four walls onto the street. It's loud, dirty, and dangerous. Fortunately, most out-of-office interactions that require treatment are near hospital care. However, it is a different situation in the unforgiving setting of the wilderness. What happens when disaster strikes during a backcountry outing and challenges your medical skills? How do you treat an ankle fracture with two protein bars, a water bottle, and a spare jacket?

The author explores the basic principles of wilderness medicine triage, survival principles, patient monitoring, and evacuation. The author also covers common and critical wilderness injuries and illnesses you may face when advanced care is hours or days away.
University of Nebraska Medical Center, 1553 Janmar Road, Snellville, GA 30078, USA
E-mail address: a-keating@att.net

Physician Assist Clin 9 (2024) 155–164
https://doi.org/10.1016/j.cpha.2023.10.001
2405-7991/24/© 2023 Elsevier Inc. All rights reserved.
physicianassistant.theclinics.com

FAST FACTS

- There are roughly 4000 to 5000 hiking-related injuries each year in the United States. The most common are falls and slips, accounting for about 50% of all accidents and injuries.[1]
- Infectious diarrhea, contact dermatitis, and tick-borne illnesses are the most common illnesses in the wilderness.[2]
- The leading cause of death for hikers more than 65 is a medical condition; myocardial infarction accounts for 36% of these fatalities.[1]
- The number one cause of death in US national parks is motor vehicle collisions, totaling 37 in 2022. It is followed closely by drownings (22 deaths) and falls/slips (22 deaths).[3]

TRIAGE PRINCIPLES

Initiating care in the wilderness using common triage principles is critical to rapid assessment, stabilization, and treatment of the patient. Triage is always relevant whether the injured are in your group or you come on an accident scene on the trail. They will help you focus your evaluation, treatment, and decision-making in the wilderness setting.[4]

Wilderness Medical Treatment

Situational evaluation

You must first evaluate the general area before any assessment or treatment of the patient can begin to avoid further harm to the patient and others. Multiple considerations are in play: weather conditions, time of day, the surrounding terrain, available supplies, and those with you. Scene evaluation has three parts: scene safety, mechanism of injury (MOI), and body substance isolation.[5]

Scene safety involves observation, evaluation, and initiation.

1. Observation: Look for loose rock, fallen trees, ground stability, safe approach, and exit pathways for those helping the patient. Also be aware of potential rapid weather changes.
2. Evaluation: Instruct those present on how to assist or ask them to leave for their safety.
3. Initiation: Use personal protective equipment (PPE) if you have it. Consider a mask for the patient in case of illnesses.[5]

Mechanism of injury is the inspection conducted once you are with the patient. The patient's position, level of consciousness, and activity can provide much information about how the injury occurred. If others are present, question whether they were witnesses. If this is an illness, quickly gather a history if possible.

Body substance isolation is taking the time to protect ourselves first with PPE. However, the easiest hand hygiene to carry with you is alcohol-based hand sanitizer, recommended over soap and water for hand sanitization.[6]

Primary patient evaluation

Before anything else, establish responsiveness. If the patient is not responsive, attempt to arouse him or her gently at first and then with painful (non-harmful) stimuli if necessary. If there is no response after several attempts, you are protected by implied consent.[7] You can proceed to your evaluation. Quickly evaluate respiratory status, circulatory stability, level of consciousness, and the need for stabilization of spinal injuries (immediately stabilize if suspected). In the wilderness, the expanded initial evaluation and treatment mnemonic are ABCDE.[8] ABC still stands for airway, breathing, and circulation. D is for decision on disability, and E is for expose and examine major injuries.[5]

Airway, breathing, and circulation evaluation is no different in the wilderness than at a local park. Perform the head-tilt–chin-lift maneuver and clear any obstructions. Check for active breathing (chest movement) and pulses over the easiest accessible artery (circulation). Provide cardiopulmonary resuscitation (CPR) to the pulseless and unresponsive patient until they are responsive or it becomes apparent that they have died. Unfortunately, in the stark reality of the wilderness, little can be done until the patient can be evacuated.

It is vital to perform a *blood sweep* (a quick gloved inspection of the patient's torso and extremities for wounds that would cause blood volume loss). Also, inspect the ground around the patient and just under the patient for additional bleeding. Apply direct pressure immediately to any wounds and elevate the limb.[5]

Decision on disability involves the neurologic assessment. It will aid in determining whether the patient is capable of transport from the immediate area to a more stable or protected area. First, determine the need for continued spinal stabilization. If the primary evaluation shows no neuro deficit or the patient states no neck pain or changes, stabilization can be discontinued. If not, or if the patient is unconscious, shore up the temporary stabilization with any available means.[5] Assessment of the patient's level of consciousness, mental status, and possible closed head injury is next. Use the APVU assessment tool: A—alert, V—voice response, P—pain response, and U—unresponsive.[8]

Expose and examine injuries is the last step. Briefly expose the skin of the extremities, looking for any missed injuries, bruising, deformities, or bites. Quickly cover to keep the patient warm.[5,8] This can be performed one limb at a time, starting with any identified areas of pain. Consider the surrounding environment and temperature and minimize the exposure time.[9] If you suspect a thoracic or abdominal trauma, ask permission to inspect the anterior torso. Posterior examination should only be conducted if there is no suspected spinal injury.

Now is the time to perform an additional scene safety appraisal. First, decide if the accident location is an appropriate place to shelter. If the area is too unstable, find the closest spot, clear a pathway, stabilize the patient (splint/make-shift stretcher), and transfer the patient to the new location. If the injury is severe and help is not forthcoming, initiate the process of sheltering in place.

No one expects to sustain or encounter an injury or illness, but knowing the basic survival skills while in the wilderness will provide the needed time to stabilize and protect the patient. The *survival rule of 3* can be applied to better understand what needs to be prioritized: You can survive for 3 minutes without air, 3 hours without shelter (in a harsh environment), 3 days without water, and 3 weeks without food.[10] Knowing this rule, the group will need to make a shelter for the patient and then themselves, obtain and purify water, gather wood, and make a fire.[11] Some sources will place food as the third priority. However, without a fire, you cannot purify the needed water or provide additional warmth.

Secondary patient evaluation

Now, advance to the secondary patient assessment, which includes a head-to-toe examination, vital signs, and medical history.

A *head-to-toe examination* is a slow, step-by-step patient examination. You will be with the patient for several hours or possibly days. Make sure to record all physical findings. Some critical physical findings may be delayed in their presentation. For example, the "Battle Sign" (ecchymosis over the mastoid process) of a basilar skull fracture may take several hours to develop, so repeat the head-to-toe examination. Recheck the splinting and look for any pressure areas due to edema. Remove the original laceration dressings. Inspect the wound, clean it as best as possible, remove contaminants, and cover it with a clean bandage.

Vital signs will need to be recorded. Follow the head-to-toe principle once more.

Head: What is their level of consciousness and responsiveness (check pupil activity)? Repeat the APVU assessment used in the primary survey and note any changes.

Chest (circulation): Monitor the heart rate, rhythm, and strength (pulses). Record the respiratory rate (breathing), effort, and breath sounds.

Temperature: Body core or temperature in the wilderness setting will likely be a tactile measurement.

Blood pressure: A palpable pulse indicates a strong enough circulation to provide blood to the extremities or normal BP. Weak or diminished distal pulses indicate poor circulation due to multiple factors (dehydration, hypovolemia, and shock).[5] Warmth of the extremities is also a good indicator, but these methods are only estimates.[12]

Medical history is the last step in the secondary assessment. Gather and record the patient's history if possible. Keep in mind that in 2022 alone, the US National Park Service recorded 17 deaths for medical reasons.[13] Even if you have done all you can do given limited supplies and location, a thorough medical history will help the next provider once the patient is evacuated.

In the event of multiple patients at an accident scene, quickly evaluate each patient using the SALT (sort, assess, lifesaving interventions, treat/transport) triage system.[14] Assign care for each patient based on the level of severity and then initiate your treatment as noted above—scene survey, primary, and secondary assessments. Be ready to accept the role of triage (medical) officer and direct the care of all the patients.[15,16]

Monitoring and evacuation

The next stage is continued care and monitoring, followed by evacuating the patient. Fortunately, with good splinting and assistance from the group, most moderately injured individuals can slowly travel to a safe destination and transportation to home or a facility. If the patient must remain in place, attempt to contact a rescue team. Talk to the group members, learn their skills, assign clear tasks according to their abilities, and check in with them often.[17]

While waiting for evacuation, continue monitoring the patient with physical checks, personal hygiene assistance, and psychological support.[5] Continue the head-to-toe checks with vitals. Hydration is more important than food. Dehydration can further complicate illnesses.

The evacuation decision can be prioritized using the same initial evaluation triage criteria.

1. *ABCDE problems*: This is the highest priority. Patients with significant airway, breathing, circulation, and shock deficits have the lowest survival rates.[18] Advanced-level care needs to be rendered as soon as possible.
2. *Neurologic problems or deficits*: The most urgent case is the person with observed or continued loss of consciousness. Next is someone showing signs and symptoms of closed head injury followed by neuro deficits of the extremities (crush injuries).[19] Crush injuries can lead to rhabdomyolysis and death due to hyperkalemia.
3. *Spinal injuries*: Spinal fractures involving spinal cord injuries (paralysis, neuro deficit, or severe pain) have high priority. Spinal injuries are very painful and require continuous immobilization to maximize a positive outcome. Fortunately, compression fractures of the vertebral bodies and laminar and transverse process fractures are relatively stable and can be treated nonsurgically.[20]

4. *Musculoskeletal trauma*: The most critical injury is an open fracture. If reduction and splinting have been achieved, the patient will need surgical intervention within 24 hours.[21] Next on the list for evacuation are those with large bone fractures as there is a high risk of neurovascular injury and compartment syndrome.[22] Stable closed fractures of the small bones, sprains, and strains can be evacuated slowly.
5. *Illnesses*: Fortunately, illness cases often respond well to rest, fluids, antipyretic medications, and time. However, patient evacuation needs increase with signs of sepsis, fever, vomiting, and/or diarrhea for more than 24 hours, dehydration or hypovolemia, or abdominal pain greater than 8 hours.[19]

Ultimately, the decision to evacuate the patient is based on the ability for you to be able to act on your decision. Complicating factors are.

- Your location (how remote)
- The other group members (how many can be sent and how fast can help be reached)
- The number of patients

Common wilderness injuries

Musculoskeletal: These injuries happen quickly, and the treatment is straightforward (strains, sprains, fractures, abrasions, and/or lacerations). Most can be treated at the scene, and the patient can often cautiously and slowly continue with the trip.

Strains, sprains, and fractures can vary from simple muscle injuries to complicated open fractures. Most of the PRICE mnemonic (Protect, Rest, Ice [if available], Compression, and Elevation) can be used. Use that spare jacket to support the stained muscle or pad the sprained ligaments. Then, secure medial and lateral bracing with any rigid splinting material (branches, rolled-up sleeping foams, parts of a backpack frame, and wood debris).[23] Be creative.

Fractures can differ significantly. Evaluate the fracture using the NOM method (Neurovascular status, Open or closed, and MOI).[24] However, in the wilderness, Displacement is an additional component (*NOM-D*). The two most important components are displacement and neurovascular status. Displaced and angulated fractures have a higher occurrence of neurovascular compromise. Reduce the fracture immediately and stabilize with padded splinting.[25] Check the neurovascular status before and after the reduction and frequently.

Most upper extremity fractures can be treated with immobilization and splinting, and the patient can self-evacuate with assistance. Post-reduction neurovascular compromise will increase the need for rapid evacuation. Use the "sling and swath" (the affected limb in a tri-corner sling with a wrap around the torso to prevent external rotation) method to immobilize after any needed reductions. Jackets work well for the swath.

Follow the same treatment protocol for lower extremity fractures. It will be the rare case where the individual can ambulate with a lower extremity fracture. Even a non-displaced distal fibula fracture is extremely painful while upright. The fracture must be stabilized (medial/lateral/posterior) with branches or firm bed rolls.[23] Next, a two-person stretcher can be fashioned from larger branches and any available material (multiple shirts, jackets, sleeping bags, tents, tarps).

The most critical fracture in any setting is an open fracture of any bone. Roughly 4% of all fractures are open.[26] Remove any clothing around the wound. Gross contamination of the wound should be irrigated with at least 1 L of treated water. You can treat a natural water source by boiling it for 5 minutes or with water purification tablets.[5] Cover with a sterile dressing or any clean clothing. If possible, the dressing should not be removed until the patient is at a higher care level.[25] A substantial infection rate increase occurs with multiple wound inspections before surgical debridement.[26] Saturated dressings may require changing.

Abrasion and laceration treatment is straightforward. Stop the bleeding—apply direct pressure and elevate the extremity. Hold until the bleeding is controlled. Clean and debride the wound—copious irrigation with treated water and sterilized pick-ups to remove embedded foreign bodies. Finally, dress the wound—air dry or pad with a fresh bandage, cover with gauze, and bulky dressing.[27]

The most serious laceration involves an arterial bleed. Direct pressure will need to be applied longer. You will need permission to use a tourniquet if it does not stop. The choice is literally "Life or Limb." A tourniquet can be placed for up to 2 hours with minimal risk of complication. However, it must be wide enough to obstruct blood flow. The minimum width is 4 cm (1.5 inches).[28] This patient will need to be evacuated on a stretcher.

Neurologic injuries range greatly. The most common neurologic complaint is headache. If there is no medical history of headaches, ask them about any trauma before or during the trip. Dehydration is a likely reason for a headache on a backpacking trip. The patient must be shaded, cooled, hydrated, and rested until the headache passes.

Closed head injury (concussion) is a common result of head trauma during a fall in the wilderness. A basic neurologic examination and simple recall of three unrelated items is a quick method to assess the severity. *"The hallmark of concussion management is absolute rest from physical and mental stimulation followed by gradual return to activity once symptoms resolve."*[29] These are the recommended guidelines for the evacuation of these patients, based on the distance needed to travel to receive advanced medical attention:

Within 1 day's travel: The patient should attempt to return with assistance, slowly, with frequent stops. Make more stops and reduce speed over rough terrain.

Within two or more days travel: Rest until symptoms improve or consider evacuating the patient. However, once the patient has gone 24 hours without symptoms, they can attempt a slow evacuation on foot. Each day, the level of exertion required can increase slightly if asymptomatic. If symptoms return, the patient must rest for 24 hours and start the restart the process, slowly advancing each day.[30]

Common wilderness illnesses

Gastrointestinal illnesses are the most common illnesses in the wilderness, followed by upper respiratory illnesses and influenza.[31] The primary treatment for gastroenteritis is prevention. Water filtration and purification is the primary prevention activity. Personal and camp hygiene is next: hand sanitizer, hand washing, proper food handling and preparation, and cleaning of cooking utensils and dinnerware. These activities will significantly decrease the risk of pathogen transmission.

Gastroenteritis can be either noninvasive or invasive. Noninvasive organisms will colonize but do not invade the lining of the intestinal walls. The released toxins cause the symptoms (cramps, nausea, vomiting, and diarrhea). Invasive organisms do breach the intestinal lining, causing dysentery. The symptoms are more severe (bloody/mucus in the stool, high fever, severe cramping, and diarrhea).[32]

The most occurring pathogen is *Giardia lamblia (water-borne protozoan), followed by Cryptosporidium (water-borne protozoan), Escherichia coli (food or water-borne bacteria), Campylobacter (food or water-borne bacteria), Salmonella (food-borne bacteria),* and *Shigella (water-borne bacteria)* are the cause of most cases of dysentery. Dysentery patients should be immediately evacuated due to the high risk of fatal outcomes and spread of the infection.[33]

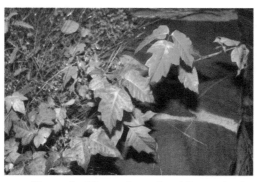

Fig. 1. Poison Ivy leaves. (Center for Disease Control and Prevention/Dr. Edwin P. Ewing Jr.)

Treatment is symptom relief and hydration. Isolate the patient from the group and practice universal precautions. Over-the-counter (OTC) Imodium (antidiarrheal) and Pepto-Bismol tablets are easy to pack and help relieve some symptoms. Dehydration prevention is the goal while the illness runs its course. Do not give antidiarrheal medications if dysentery is suspected. Rest and rehydrate the patient until they are stable.[34]

Upper respiratory illnesses will be treated symptomatically in the same manner as gastroenteritis. Isolate the patient, universal precautions, rest, fluids, and, if available— antipyretics, antihistamines, and decongestants.[35] They can advance after not having a fever for 24 hours.

Most wilderness contact dermatitis is due to poison ivy or poison oak. Know what both look like (**Fig. 1**).

Warn the group when observed and treat the rash with topical corticosteroids and OTC topical preparations (**Fig. 2**).[36]

Tick-borne illnesses can be reduced with the application of insect repellants. Otherwise, properly remove the tick, wash the bite area, and observe the patient. Have the individual inform you of any classic rash (spotted or bullseye), fever, muscle cramping, or arthralgias.[5]

Practical preparation

Wilderness medicine is often austere medicine. Most people do not venture outdoors with a full medic pack ready for any eventuality. We go to our destinations, lock the car, throw on our backpacks with water bottles, and start hiking. What can we take in our backpack to help us care for an injury that won't take up our entire bag?

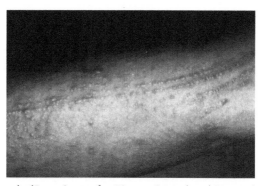

Fig. 2. Poison Oak rash. (*From* Center for Disease Control and Prevention.)

First aid kit: how to choose a kit

Anyone who has ever walked more than an hour in the woods on changing terrain knows that the more you carry, the more it weighs. There are a multitude of first aid packs available for purchase. They range from adhesive bandages and triple antibiotic ointment to complete trauma kits. It can be overwhelming choosing one. Here are some questions to ask yourself when purchasing your first aid pack.

1. How much do I want to spend?
2. How much do I want to carry (weight of the kit)?
3. How long will I be gone (trip length)?
4. How many people are in the group?

I prefer to review a kit content list and build my kit to save money and take what I need. It is up to you to know what you need based on your experience and skill level. Pack what you know and know what you packed.

SUMMARY

Wilderness medicine injuries and illness can occur 6 minutes, 6 miles, or 6 days into a backcountry adventure. Most injuries and illnesses are easy to treat, and the person can continue their trip. We have the added responsibility of knowing how to provide care for those in our group or those we might meet on the trail. The assessment principle of ABCDE aids and focuses on the rapid assessment and examination of the patient. The wilderness setting requires us to quickly prioritize our treatment decisions, especially if we have more than one patient. The challenge for the non-wilderness medicine clinician knows how to care for a patient with minimal resources.

CLINICS CARE POINTS

- Be ready to assume the role of the medical expert in the event of an injury or illness in the wilderness.
- Approach every patient assessment in the same manner using the ABCDE mnemonic.
- Wilderness medical treatment involves rapid assessment, stabilization, essential first aid/treatment, and evacuation.
- Follow the principles of situational evaluation, primary patient evaluation, and secondary patient evaluation to maximize the survivability of your patient in the wilderness setting.

DISCLOSURE

There is no financial relationship with any commercial interest related to the article's content. This article was solely researched and developed by the author.

REFERENCES

1. Martirosian D. 33 troubling hiking injury and death statistic. Hikers Daily; 2022. Available at. https://hikersdaily.com/hiking-injury-statistics/. Accessed 26 August, 2023.
2. Harsant S. Top 5 Wilderness Medicine Topics for the Urgent Care Provider. Journal of Urgent Care Medicine 2019. Available at. https://www.jucm.com/top-5-wilderness-medicine-topics-for-the-urgent-care-provider/. Accessed 26 August, 2023.

3. News Nation On the Go Staff Authors. More than 200 people died in national parks last year: These were the deadliest. April 27, 2023. Available at https://www.newsnationnow.com/us-news/more-than-200-people-died-in-national-parks-last-year-these-were-the-deadliest/, Accessed 26 August, 2023.

4. Nakao H, Ukai I, Kotani J. A review of the history of the origin of triage from a disaster medicine perspective. Acute Medicine and Surgery 2017;4(4):379–84.

5. Tod Schiemelpfenig. NOLS wilderness medicine. 7th ed. Guiford, CT: Stackpole Books; 2021. p. 3–7, 9, 12-18, 20, 23-25, 282.

6. Khairar MR, Anintha G, Dalvi TM, et al. Comparative Efficacy of Hand Disinfection Potential of Hand Sanitizer and Liquid Soap among Dental Students: A Randomized Controlled Trial. Indian J Crit Care Med 2020;24(5):336–9.

7. Richards EP. The Climate Change and Public Health Law Site, LSU law center, Emergency Exception, https://biotech.law.lsu.edu/books/aspen/Aspen-THE- 11. html, Accessed 26 August, 2023.

8. Thim T, Krarup NHV, Grove EL, et al. Initial assessment and treatment with the Airway, Breathing, Circulation, Disability, Exposure (ABCDE) approach. Int J Gen Med 2012;5:117–21.

9. Staff Writers. Emergency Care and First Aid for the Outdoors and Travel: The ABCD's of Emergency Care. Italiaoutdoors. https://www.italiaoutdoors.com/index.php/first-aid-planning/569- outdoors-skills/first-aid-outdoors/first-aid-planning/624-the-abc d-s-of-emergency-care, Accessed 26 August, 2023.

10. Staff Writers. Wilderness Survival Rule of 3 – Air, Shelter, Water and Food. BackcountryChronicles.com. 2011-2023. https://www.backcountrychronicles.com/wilderness-survival-rules-of-3/, Accessed 26August2023.

11. Hwang V. Four Needs of Wilderness Survival. Trackers Earth. https://trackersearth.com/blog/four-needs-of-wilderness-survival, Accessed 26August2023.

12. Iverson K, Donner HJ. Improvised Medicine in the Wilderness: Chapter 23. Emerg Med 2016. Available at. https://aneskey.com/improvised-medicine-in-the-wilderness/. Accessed 26 August, 2023.

13. Hysi I. National Park Service Excel Spread Sheet. NPS Mortality Data CY2007-CY2023, Released April 2023. https://www.google.com/search?q=NPS+mortality+'" for+CY+2007-2023& rlz=1C1CHBF_enUS1010US1010& oq=NPS+mortality+'" for+CY+2007-2023& aqs=chrome.69i57.15302j0j7& sourceid=chrome& ie=UTF-8, Accessed 26 August, 2023.

14. Cone DC, Serra J, Burns K, et al. Pilor test of the SALT mass casualty triage system. Prehosp Emerg Care 2009;13(4):536–40.

15. DeNolf RL, Kahwaji CI. EMS Mass Casualty Management. 2022 Oct 10. In: StatPearls [internet]. Treasure Island (FL: StatPearls Publishing; 2023.

16. Staff Writers. Medical Professionals - Trauma. Mass casualty triage guidelines revised. Mayo Clinic On-line. May 08, 2021. https://www.mayoclinic.org/medical-professionals/trauma/news/mass-casualty-triage-guidelines-revised/mac-20512735, Accessed 26 August, 2023

17. Hogwood C. Key Roles and Team Dynamics Within the Survival Group. Survival Dispatch. January 20, 2020. https://survivaldispatch.com/key-roles-and-team-dynamics-within-the-survival-group/, Accessed 26August2023.

18. Park, A, Seibert T. Force of Nature - Trauma in the Wilderness, Lesson 6. Critical Decisions in Emergency Medicine March 2019 Volume 33 Number 3, https://www.acep.org/siteassets/sites/acep/media/sections/wilderness/wilderness-trauma-cdem-article.pdf, Accessed 28August2023.

19. McEvoy D, Moore G, Bleicher J et al. Wilderness Medicine, 14th Edition. Missoula, MT. Ryan Milling, 2019. Page 110-111, http://aeriemedicine.com/uploads/

documents/Aerie%2014th%20Edition%20Manual%20PDF%20Final.pdf, Accessed 28 August, 2023.

20. Park D. Diseases and Conditions: Fractures of the Thoracic and Lumbar Spine. OrthoInfo On-line. AAOS, June 2020. https://orthoinfo.aaos.org/en/diseases-conditions/fractures-of-the-thoracic-and-lumbar-spine/, Accessed 29August2023.

21. Srour M, Inaba K, Okoye O, et al. Prospective evaluation of treatment of open fractures: effect of time to irrigation and debridement. JAMA Surg 2015;150(4): 332–6.

22. Elliott KG, Johnstone AJ. Diagnosing acute compartment syndrome. J Bone Joint Surg Br 2003;85(5):625–32.

23. O'Connor T. Splinting Review. University of Colorado – Section of Wilderness and Environmental Medicine, Department of Emergency Medicine On-line. Aurora, Colorado, https://www.coloradowm.org/blog/splinting-review/, Accessed 28August 2023.

24. Keating, A. Orthopedic Emergencies: The Common and the Critical. Physician Assistant Clinics, https://www.sciencedirect.com/science/article/abs/pii/S2405799123000543.

25. Quinn RH, Macias DJ. The management of open fractures. Wilderness Environ Med 2006;17(1):41–8.

26. Court-Brown CM, McQueen MM, Quaba AA. Management of open fractures. London, UK: Martin Dunitz; 1996.

27. Harper B. Wilderness Wound Care. Drivers Alert Network. February 1, 2010, https://dan.org/alert-diver/article/wilderness-wound-care/, Accessed 30August2023.

28. Quinn RH, Wedmore I, Johnson E, et al. Wilderness Medical Society practice guidelines for basic wound management in the austere environment. Wilderness Environ Med 2014;25(3):295–310.

29. McCrory P, Meeuwisse WH, Aubry M, et al. Consensus statement on concussion in sport: the 4th International Conference on Concussion in Sport held in Zurich, November 2012. Br J Sports Med 2013;47(5):250–8.

30. Wright JM, Islas AA. Concussion management in the wilderness. Wilderness Environ Med 2014;25(3):319–24.

31. McIntosh SE, Leemon D, Visitacion J, et al. Medical incidents and evacuations on wilderness expeditions. Wilderness Environ Med 2007 Winter;18(4):298–304.

32. Tilton B. Backcountry Diarrhea: Treating the Runs. Outside. October 1, 1997. https://www.backpacker.com/skills/backcountry-diarrhea-treating-the-runs/, Accessed 1September2023.

33. Center for Disease Control and Prevention, A Guide to Drinking Water Treatment and Sanitation for Backcountry and Travel Use. 20Jul2023. https://www.cdc.gov/healthywater/drinking/travel/backcountry_water_treatment.html, Accessed 1September2023.

34. Staff Authors. How to Treat Waterborne Illness in the Backcountry. Appalachian Mountain Club. 27Feb2020, https://www.outdoors.org/resources/amc-outdoors/outdoor-resources/how-to-treat-waterborne-illness-in-the-backcountry/, 2September 2023.

35. Buer S. What To Do If You Get Sick While Camping. NOLS Blog On-line, 12Jan2017, https://blog.nols.edu/2017/01/13/how-to-handle-flu-like-illness-in-the-backcountry, 5September2023.

36. Auxier, G. Your guide to treating illness or injury in the great outdoors. Contemporary Pediatrics. 1May2015, https://www.contemporarypediatrics.com/view/wilderness-medicine-your-guide-treating-illness-or-injury-great-outdoors, 6September2023.

Military Medicine Outside Four Walls

Rodney Ho, PhD, MPAS, MPH, PA-C, Psychiatry-CAQ[a],*,
Derrick Varner, PhD, PA-C, DFAAPA, RDMS[b],
Jason Pearce Beissinger, MS, PA-C, DiMM[c]

KEYWORDS

- Military medicine • War medicine • Air force PA • Army PA • Navy PA

KEY POINTS

- Military medicine has been the source of a huge number of medical innovations, from tourniquets to triage to ambulances to prosthetics to organ transplants.
- Each military service has unique medical capabilities based on their mission and environment (sea, land, air, and/or space) of responsibility.
- PAs in the military perform a full range of services from OB to pediatrics to adult medicine to psychiatry.

INTRODUCTION

From the beginning of time, opposing sides have taken to battle for supremacy. Where there is conflict, there is injury and the need for treatment. Texts from Egypt, 1600 BCE, describe wound care, splinting of fractures, and the use of cauterization for bleeding. When the ancient Babylonian Assyrians went to battle, their physician-priests cast the necessary spells and performed ritual magic, but they also had "asu," the first full-time military physicians.

Roman military medicine has much in common with practice today. The practitioners understood sanitation and designed camps to protect the water supply and locate latrines downstream from drinking water. Unfortunately, much of what the Romans practiced was lost during the Middle Ages and practitioners often based treatments on humors and astrology. Some historians believe that the latter is one reason we collect patients' date of birth. Medical care of the wounded was left to servants and camp followers. In other words, the wounded were pretty much on their own.

[a] Rocky Mountain University, UT, USA; [b] MA, USA; [c] Portland Mountain Rescue, Happy Valley, OR, USA
* Corresponding author.
E-mail address: horodney26@gmail.com

Physician Assist Clin 9 (2024) 165–173
https://doi.org/10.1016/j.cpha.2023.10.002
2405-7991/24/Published by Elsevier Inc.

physicianassistant.theclinics.com

Ambrose Pare´, a barber surgeon, is credited with reviving Roman battlefield medicine. He used turpentine as an antiseptic, applied ligatures to tie off bleeding vessels, and invented hemostats. The eighteenth century saw great advances with the invention of tourniquets and forceps to remove bullets and fragments. This period also saw the publication of books on military medicine.[1]

With war comes progress; Mary Merritt Crawford, the only woman physician at the American Hospital during World War I, stated: "A war benefits medicine more than it benefits anybody else. It's terrible, of course, but it does."[2] The Napoleonic wars brought us the concept of triage and carriages designated for removing the wounded from front lines.[1]

US MILITARY

When one thinks of "medicine outside four walls,"military medicine, practiced in the field, in tents or in third world countries, often comes to mind. Medicine in the military is often at remote sites with limited supplies, and the military practitioners are known for their daring and inventive ideas. Often this is under the extreme circumstance of war. We first saw use of dialysis machines during the Korean War.[3] Nursing and Florence Nightingale caring for patients in the field are intrinsically intertwined. Jonathan Letterman, MD, a Union Army physician, has been called the "Father of Modern Battlefield Medicine" for his many contributions. He is credited with the first organized ambulance service and established a triage of three levels of field hospital care. Amputations using ether were performed during the Civil War. Prosthetics used in this century are all based on designs from those developed by the military. Organ transplant surgery, plastic surgery, ambulances, tourniquets, blood collection and donation, and trauma medicine all have their roots in military medicine.[3,4] A significant amount of the expertise of search and rescue, high-altitude transport, helicopter medevac rescue, and/or cave and scuba rescue are due to the experience of military medicine.[4] With all that military medicine has contributed to civilian medicine, it is discouraging to realize that few civilians know or comprehend the incredible contributions of our military forces. In 2021, the US Census reports less than 10% of the population have any military overlap.[5] Yet, it is impossible to discuss wilderness or austere medicine without first understanding military medicine.

There are six branches of the military (Marines, Navy, Army, Air Force, Space Force, and Coast Guard), and each has an assigned medical corp. The Coast Guard is not a formal military branch but is instead under Homeland Security. The Navy supplies the medical care for the Marines. All military branches function under a "tooth and tail" set up, tooth referring to the combat troops and tail referring to the logistics support for the tooth. Each branch has a different layout for tooth and tail; that is, in the Army, it is 30% tooth and 70% tail. In the Air Force, it is 10% tooth and 90% tail. Military medicine is considered part of the "tail."

The qualifications and titles of the military medical corps depend on the service. Within the Army, historically medics are often trained "on the job," attached to a particular infantry group and are expected to care for the soldiers in their division. This can be as simple as treating colds, pains, or strains to as complicated as evaluating a soldier while under fire in a combat zone. Medics are the backbone of military medicine and are the most likely to be practicing medicine in the field. There is little doubt why this group was the first to be integrated into the new "PA profession" by Dr Eugene Stead, Jr.[6]

The creation of the first phyisican assistant (PA) program in the Air Force was under a directive from Lieutenant General (Lt Gen) Alanzo A Towner.[7] Lt Gen Towner is considered to the "Godfather of the PA program" with the initial PA program at Sheppard Air Force Base (AFB) in Wichita Falls, TX.[7] The first class of PAs graduated in 1971 as enlisted personnel, although at present time, PAs are commissioned officers.[7] Specialty PAs (general surgery, orthopedics, and otolaryngology) were followed by the first emergency medicine PA fellowship (1991) developed at Los Angeles County Hospital. In 1995, the first Air Force PA was placed in Special Operations aeromedical division. The Army developed a PA program at Ft Sam Houston with the first graduating class in 1973. An Interservice PA program (IPAP) was opened in 1996, and all military branches were enrolled. IPAP is still the main training site for all military PAs, all branches.[7]

In the Army, there are four levels of health care. An Army medic is assigned to an infantry unit (first level) but if more care is needed, the injured soldier is moved to a battalion aid station (second level). These are often manned by PAs and can be very austere and near the fighting. A third level of Army combat care is a combat support hospital (**Fig. 1**)

This is the type of medical unit that is depicted in the series mobile army surgical hospital (MASH) and is behind front lines but can also be moved if needed. The fourth level of care is a major hospital system (ie, *Landstuhl in Germany or Brian Allgood Army Community Hospital in Korea*) and the Air Force will be used to medevac the patient to the site (**Fig. 2**).

The Air Force was established in 1947 as a separate entity from the Army.[8] Initially, the Army was mandated to provide all health care-related services for the Air Force, but in 1949, the Secretary of the Defense formed an Air Force Medical Service (AFMS).[8] The AFMS consisted of the Medical Corps, Dental Corps, Nurse Corps, Veterinary Corps, Medical Service Corps, and Women's Medical Specialist Corps. This morphed into a separate Biomedical Sciences Corp with 17 allied health specialties, from bioenvironmental engineers to occupational/physical therapists to public health officers, psychologists, social workers, pharmacists, optometrists, and PAs among others.

The Air Force has four medical fellowships for experienced PAs (emergency medicine, general surgery, orthopedic surgery, and otolaryngology), or they can move into administration. PAs in the medical fellowships are trained at the Brooke Army Medical Center, although their degree will be granted by Baylor University. After several years of practice and meeting certain requirements, if one desires, they can apply for one of the highly competitive fellowship programs.

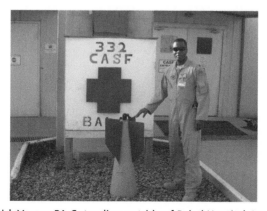

Fig. 1. Major Derrick Varner, PA-C standing outside of Balad Hospital, Iraq. Largest hospital in Iraq, trauma level III. (Used with permission Derrick Varner.)

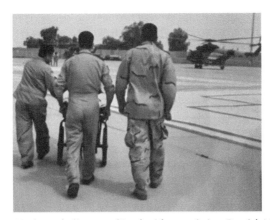

Fig. 2. Transport to Medevac helicopter. (Used with permission Derrick Varner.)

In addition, there are opportunities for Air Force PAs to attend a Flight Medicine course at Wright Patterson AFB, OH (fixed-wing) or Fort Rucker Army Base, AL (rotatory wing). Rotatory wing aircraft are used more intra-theater and fixed-wing aircraft can be used both intra-theater and intercontinental to transport injured, emergent, or critically ill patients. At times, a deployed Air Force PA may be assigned to a medevac helicopter unit used to transport injured military personnel. A Black Hawk helicopter (rotatory wing) can hold six stretchers and four ambulatory patients. The larger planes (fixed-wing) are designed to evacuate larger groups of injured military or civilian patients on a C-141 and C-5 (**Fig. 3**).

These larger airplanes are used for more distance transport to the regional hospital systems once patients are stable enough for transport. The Air Force has a specialized team: "Critical Care Air Transport Team," composed of trained physicians, nurses, and respiratory therapists to manage the transfer patient(s) and literally have a "mini-intensive care unit" (ICU) that sits above the stretchers for the most unstable patients. If managing an ICU patient in a military transport aircraft in the middle of the ocean is not "austere" medicine, then nothing is.

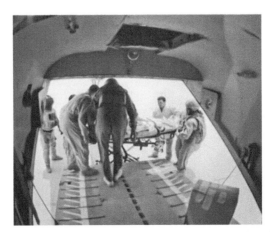

Fig. 3. Unloading patient from the rotatory wing aircraft to a stretcher. (Used with permission from Derrick Varner.)

As the only medical service in a distant outpost, often the military medical providers will also care for the local population and detainees. In Iraq, a PA was responsible for the medical care of the detainees who were jailed as "enemy combatants." Although he was in a distant outpost housed in a cement block building with minimal equipment, the medical care he rendered was often the first that many of these combatants had ever received. He reports that he diagnosed multiple cases of diabetes and hypertension but was most impressed by the "tetralogy of Fallot" that he found in adults. He operated with very limited supplies; he had a spin-crit, a stethoscope, a glucometer, and some medications. He was also responsible for the medical care of the military police who manned the jail.

Another PA reports that while stationed at an Afghanistan trauma site, she found that she was mainly diagnosing and treating the locals rather than the soldiers she had expected. An Army MASH unit, surgical tech spoke of the adjustments that had to be made during the hot, windy days when posted to the desert. Because the whipping sand would get into the anesthesia machines and the heat of the daytime increased the wind, there was no way to keep patients anesthetized safely for surgery. Attempts were made to "sand-proof" the tents but that made the inside of the sites too hot for work. By converting to nighttime surgery, they were able to manage the patients and keep the medical staff safe. One of the authors spent significant time training Iraqi nationals on triage care for evacuation (**Figs. 4** and **5**).

As the worldwide politics change and adapt, so does military medicine. Many of these practitioners are now working in and/or managing clinics whose population is mainly dependents, retirees, children, and spouses of the active-duty troops. The large military hospital residency programs have also had to adjust to a different patient mix. The Camp Pendleton family practice residency was put on notice because it did not have enough "chronic conditions" for the residents to manage. Although the residents were experts on pregnancy and delivery along with orthopedics (this is a Marine outpost), there were no patients with diabetes or hypertension. Often having a chronic disease will mean separation from the military. By adding management of retirees and families, the residency program stayed viable.[9]

Training for medical care for the troops often means that one is dealing with teenagers who are away from home for the first time. Many of these troops are 17 to 18 year old and have never seen the ocean, let alone tried to swim in 65° water (Camp Pendleton in San Diego). The medical staff at the large intake bases are experts

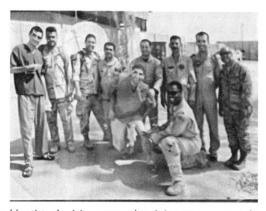

Fig. 4. Iraqi Medics (dentist, physicians, nurses) training on transport. (Used with permission from Derrick Varner.)

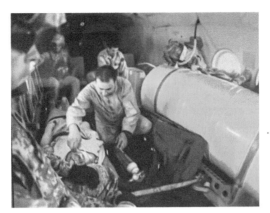

Fig. 5. Providing instructions to Iraqi Medics providing care in flight. (Used with permission from Derrick Varner.)

in alcohol poisoning, homesickness, and sexually transmitted diseases. The physical training of the Navy physicians that will care for the Marines is often done during the summer at Camp Pendleton (west coast) or Camp Lejeune (east coast). Summer entertainment on these bases includes watching big, gruff, loud, well-conditioned Marine drill sergeants trying to corral a group of nerdy looking doctor recruits into shape- …whereas the docs stop to vomit every so often during "physical conditioning."

When Navy PAs are first trained, they are sent to a hospital, clinic, Marine unit, or more likely, a small ship (ie, an oiler vs an Air Craft Carrier) as the chief medical officer. Although the military spends a significant amount of time on medical issues, including tropical diseases, they also train their medical staff for psychiatric management. PAs report that as they suture wounds or x-ray chests, the young recruits may talk of homesickness, family issues, and sometimes suicide. The medical staff has specialized training in post-traumatic stress disorders (PTSD) as the frequency of this diagnosis in the military is higher than in civilians. PTSD has its roots in the evaluation of soldiers from multiple wars, from the Civil War to the Vietnam War. PTSD was first introduced in the psychiatric *Diagnostic and Statistical Manual of Mental Disorders* (DSM 3rd Edition) in 1980 to describe and classify experiences of patients, mainly Vietnam War veterans.[10] PTSD has been studied extensively with war veterans and is synonymous with other previous wartime diagnoses: shell shock, stress syndrome, battle fatigue, or traumatic war neurosis.[11] Military medics have specialized training in combat stress and PTSD due to the high prevalence of these mental health diagnosis secondary to deployment and wartime experiences. Owing to the increase in need, in 2020, the Department of Defense (DoD) Psychiatric PA fellowship was created and the first DoD Psychiatric PA graduated in 2021.[12] These mental health care experts care for military members traumatized by stresses ranging from COVID-19 to war to overseas postings.

Within the Air Force National Guard, PAs and nurse practitioner (NP) participate in the *Chemical/Biological/Radiation/Nuclear/Explosive Enhances Response Force Package* (CERFP) in military parlance. These units each exist within one of the ten Federal Emergency Management Agency (FEMA) zones of the United States. These units are responsible for providing technical and medical resources in the event of a disaster. The CERFP units typically compose of units for.

- Search and extraction

- Ambulatory patient stabilization
- Non-ambulatory patient stabilization
- Triage
- Command staff leadership

CERFP units work in hazardous material and disaster environments. They are highly mobile and deployed to an area to quickly establish a "footprint" to facilitate their mission. Search and extraction teams may be responsible for high-angle patient access and field care. After bringing the patient to a decontamination zone, the triage process starts. Patients are grouped by acuity and then moved through the various treatment area tents for initial stabilization. Last, patients are processed and transferred to available local community medical care sites such as hospitals or other established resources.

Within these unique units, PAs/NPs may function as field care providers, command and control staff, and/or training officers. While often employed in patient care, PAs/NPs have served at the highest level of leadership roles. Similar to other military roles, theirs is a unique cultural blend of medical hierarchy and military rank, which must be homogenized to effectively carry out the unit mission.

MEDICAL RESERVE CORPS

After 9/11, the "Medical Reserve Corps" (MRC) network was established.[13] Based on military medicine and hierarchy, the MRC has more than 300,000 volunteer medical experts that can be called up by the state when a large influx of experts is needed. Each state is responsible for the recruitment, training, and choice of activation for their local MRCs. All MRCs follow the *National Incident Management* structure developed by Homeland Security. This allows for easy integration of MRCs across state lines, within the state, national, and federal emergency rescue system, including FEMA.

The MRCs are set-up before the need for their activation. Any medical professional can contact their county or state emergency experts. MRCs will do the vetting of the volunteer before the need. This usually requires a background check, license certification, and training to allow incident commander planning during an emergency. Free online training and certification for incident management are available on the Homeland Security Web site.[14] MRCs have been activated in California to manage those civilians evacuated during fires or earthquakes, Florida to staff sites for those displaced by hurricanes, NJ for those affected by flooding, Puerto Rico for hurricanes, Texas for vet services during hurricane flooding, and multiple states for emergency care, search and rescue, or simply vaccination clinics during a pandemic. MRCs are a way for the practitioner to give back to their community while simultaneously practicing medicine outside four walls.

SUMMARY

Military medicine and "Medicine outside 4 Walls" are synonymous. The civilian medical community has much to thank military medicine for, from nursing to ambulances to tourniquets to blood banks and more. The military medical community has learned to work together by delegating jobs between all branches, producing excellent medical care in high-stress situations. Military medicine can also be one of the best diplomatic/political outreaches the United States has to offer. Although many know and accept the medical expertise of the military, the logistical expertise of military medicine is just as useful. The formal adoption of the MRC for civilian medicine during a crisis has shown us that especially, in times of emergencies. As always, the military has played a large role in creating and sustaining the PA profession.

CLINICS CARE POINTS

- Military medicine is responsible for much of the explosion of medical care development in the twentieth century.
- The Navy has expertise in medicine at sea; the Air Force has expertise in flight medicine and medical transfer of patients, whereas the Army has expertise in medicine on land.
- The logistical organization developed by the military has been adapted by non-military emergency services with excellent results.

DISCLOSURE

With special thanks to Robert Glasgow IV (LCDR Medical Service Corp, Navy), Alan Abrams (Army Medical Corp), and others who contributed to this article. The authors would also thank them for their service. The views and written materials expressed in this publication do not necessarily represent the views of the United States Air Force, Department of Defense and/or the United States Government.

REFERENCES

1. VanWay CW. War and Trauma: A history of military medicine. Mo Med 2016;260: 113–4.
2. Hampton E, How World War I Revolutionized Medicine, https://www.theatlantic.com/health/archive/2017/02/world-war-i-medicine/517656/Accessed 27Jul2023.
3. Zuber K, Ho R. The Secret Side of the Military and the Kidney. Physician Assist Clin 2022;7:347–56.
4. Samuel L. 6 medical innovations that moved from the battlefield to mainstream medicine, 10Nov2017, https://www.statnews.com/2017/11/10/medical-innovations-war/.
5. Schaeffer K. The changing face of America's veteran population-Census Bureau Releases New Report on Veterans, www.pewresearch.org/fact-tank/2021/04/05/the-changing-face-of-americas-veteran-population/, Accessed 27Jul 2023.
6. Miller, L. The birth of the Physician Assistant. 15Nov2016, Smithsonian special exhibits, https://circulatingnow.nlm.nih.gov/2016/11/15/the-birth-of-the-physician-assistant/, Accessed 8Aug2023.
7. Tuttle, D.W. (n.d.). More Than a Nurse, Less Than a Doctor: A History of Physician Assistants Training. Office of History, 82D Training Wing, Sheppard AFB, Air Education and Training Command.
8. National Museum of the United States Air Force, USAF fact sheet, https://www.nationalmuseum.af.mil/Visit/Museum-Exhibits/Fact-Sheets/Display/Article/195791/usaf-established/, Accessed 8Aug2023.
9. Personal communication, Kim Zuber, PA-C Fall, Camp Pendleton, CA, 2015.
10. American Psychiatric Association (APA). Diagnostic and statistical manual of mental disorders. 3rd edition. Washington, DC: American Psychiatric Publishing; 1980.
11. Jones JA. From nostalgia to post-traumatic stress disorder: A mass society theory of psychological reactions to combat. Int Student J 2013;05(2):1–3.

12. US Department of Veteran's Affairs, Physician Assistant Post-graduate Residency in Mental Health, https://www.va.gov/houston-health-care/work-with-us/internships-and-fellowships/physician-assistant-post-graduate-residency-in-mental-health/, Accessed 8 August, 2023.
13. Dept of Health and Human Services, Administration for Strategic Preparedness and Response, https://aspr.hhs.gov/MRC/Pages?index.aspx, Accessed 27July, 2023.
14. FEMA First Response Training, National Training and Education Division, https://www.firstrespondertraining.gov/frts/npcc, Accessed 27 July, 2023.

Street Medicine

Brandon R. Beattie, MMSc, PA-C*, Fatima Elgarguri, BS, PA/MPH-S

KEYWORDS

- Street medicine • Mobile medicine • Health disparities • Population health
- Homeless

KEY POINTS

- Street Medicine practitioners carry supplies and medications on foot to deliver healthcare to patients.
- Mobile Medicine practitioners provide healthcare to patients wherever they are via Mobile Health Clinics.
- Street Medicine and Mobile Medicine care modalities help deliver high-quality, cost-effective healthcare to highly vulnerable populations.

INTRODUCTION

Street Medicine (SM), a term initially coined by Dr James Withers in 1992, is defined as providing care directly to unhoused people where they live, both on the street and in shelters.[1,2] Homeless individuals often lack access to traditional healthcare services due to financial constraints, stigma, and mental health challenges.[3] Without primary care, they often end up in hospital emergency rooms with multiple advanced health issues. By meeting people where they are, often in encampments, parks, or under bridges, SM practitioners aim to provide care to those who might otherwise face difficulty accessing treatment.[4] The goal is to address the preventable morbidity and mortality that occurs when these vulnerable populations slip through the cracks of traditional fixed-site healthcare settings.[5]

While SM as a formal movement is relatively new, reaching people on their own terms harkens back to one of the earliest methods of practicing medicine: the house call. Until the mid-20th century, the classic image of a clinician was that of a general practitioner, medical bag in hand, traveling to a patient's home where they would provide care.[6] The house call has gone out of fashion due to systematic changes in medical technology. Yet it does live on in the form of SM through the upheld value of creating a therapeutic alliance by recognizing the patient's specific needs within their

The George Washington University, Department of PA Studies, School of Medicine and Health Sciences, Watergate Office Building, 2600 Virginia Avenue NW, Suite 120, Washington, DC, USA
* Corresponding author.
E-mail address: bbeattie@gwu.edu

Physician Assist Clin 9 (2024) 175–185
https://doi.org/10.1016/j.cpha.2023.11.002
2405-7991/24/© 2023 Elsevier Inc. All rights reserved.

physicianassistant.theclinics.com

lived context. This alliance is critical in the context of the precarious living conditions often faced by individuals experiencing homelessness. Just as house calls provide personalized care to patients, healthcare providers practicing SM aim to provide holistic care that considers the whole person and their circumstances.

SM and mobile medicine (MM) can help fill the gaps where the mainstream healthcare delivery model fails to meet the needs of unhoused or under-resourced populations. On any given night in the United States, an estimated 200,000 people are sleeping on the streets, and an additional 400,000 are sleeping in homeless shelters.[7] People experiencing homelessness have a shortened lifespan, nearly three decades shorter than their housed counterparts. Often, these early deaths are due to preventable medical conditions. The all-cause mortality rate of the unhoused is 5 to 10 times higher than the general population.[8,9] However, these patients face multiple barriers to accessing healthcare in traditional settings, including financial, transportation difficulties, and stigma associated with homelessness. This leads to a distrust of the medical environment.[3] SM and MM provide a socially responsible alternative to overcome such obstacles and meet the needs of these vulnerable populations.

SM programs typically offer the same primary care services obtained in physical clinics, from basic wound care and vaccinations to perinatal care to managing chronic illnesses (including hypertension, diabetes, human immunodeficiency virus, etc.) while also providing mental healthcare.[10,11] Practitioners carrying backpacks filled with supplies and medications meet their patients where they are.[10] Practitioners can also appropriately triage conditions requiring immediate treatment and help connect patients to emergency services. In addition to delivering medical assistance, SM practitioners often collaborate with social service organizations, housing agencies, and harm reduction specialists.[5,12] The emphasis is on providing essential medical services and addressing the complex social determinants of health contributing to the patients' vulnerable situations (**Fig. 1**).

Mobile Medicine

Similar to SM, MM helps deliver care to highly vulnerable populations wherever the patients are but practices out of mobile health clinics (MHCs) rather than backpacks. The patient populations can include those experiencing homelessness, the uninsured, veterans, and/or immigrants.[13] In addition to vulnerable populations, commercial MM companies have begun to provide healthcare to patients with health insurance, the elderly, people with transportation difficulties or disabilities, or those

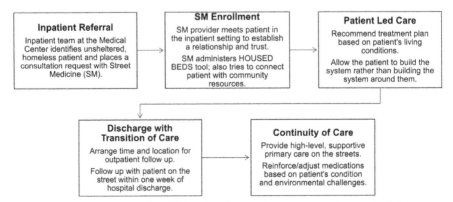

Fig. 1. Street medicine workflow.[12] (Used with permission - Laura Mosqueda, MD.)

with economic means capable of paying cash for visits.[14] Rather than being limited by the number of supplies one can carry on their persons, healthcare providers practicing MM have more abundant resources and supplies to utilize when rendering aid. As of 2023, an estimated 2000 MHCs were currently operating in the United States (**Fig. 2**).[11,15]

MHCs are most effective in providing services such as urgent care, primary care, preventative screenings, and initiating management and lifestyle modifications for chronic diseases.[11] Specialty care can include dental, mammography, and ophthalmology screenings.[11] Providers who practice medicine from these mobile clinics are often strongly motivated to help underserved community members.[10,17] MHCs help reduce barriers to healthcare, including time, transportation logistics, and navigation of the complex US healthcare industry.[13] MM continues to be an underutilized medium for delivering high-quality, cost-effective care to patients who may otherwise not seek treatment (**Table 1**).[18]

SM clinicians offer medical services on foot, differentiating this type of care from MM where services are provided from a vehicle setting. For many SM providers, this divergence in care delivery intentionally upholds the goal of minimizing the power imbalance between patients and providers. Despite this philosophic distinction, SM and MM can be considered complementary services along the same continuum. Both methods directly engage with patients in their familiar environments and foster personal connections and rapport that aim to transcend societal biases and patient transportation challenges. Many providers practice in both settings, and the delivery method can vary based on what the patient population calls for that day. There are nuanced variations with each approach (see **Table 1**). For example, mobile clinics can offer the advantage of more specialized services compared to SM. However, SM may be more successful in certain areas where mobile clinics struggle with access or engagement, and vice versa. Ultimately, the *"best fit"* type of program depends on the financial resources, geographic reach, and unique needs of each population served.

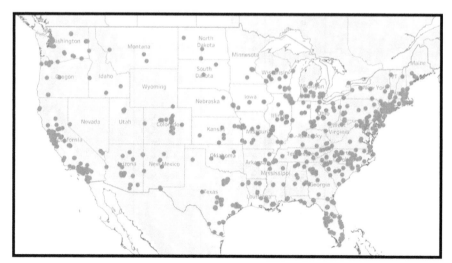

Fig. 2. Mobile health clinics operating in the United States of America.[16] Each orange marker represents a mobile clinic. An interactive map may be found at https://www. mobilehealthmap.org/find-clinics/. (Used with permission - Mollie Williams, DrPH, MPH.)

Table 1
Comparing and contrasting street medicine with mobile medicine[10,11,13,17,18]

	Description of Healthcare Delivery	Advantages	Types of Care	Ethos	Payment
Street Medicine	Backpack medicine providing direct care in the places patients reside	Agility/ability to access hard-to-reach areas Lack of mobile unit repair costs	Urgent care, primary care, minimal preventative care	Motivated by commitment to underserved communities Emphasis on suspending traditional patient-provider hierarchy	Public insurance, private insurance, philanthropy, federal grants, cash-payments
Mobile Medicine	Medicine provided from a customized vehicle Go to places patients reside	Capacity for expanded services	Urgent care, primary care, preventative care, dental work	Motivated by a commitment to underserved communities	Public insurance, private insurance, philanthropy, federal grants, cash-payments

DISCUSSION

The impact of the COVID-19 pandemic on people experiencing homelessness cannot be understated. Living in communal living spaces, both formal and informal, without regular access to running water, this setting is ripe for the transmission of communicable diseases such as COVID-19.[8] Coupled with increased difficulties adhering to Center for Disease Control and Prevention (CDC) policies for reducing the transmission of COVID-19, the unsheltered were among the highest at-risk populations.[19] A novel 2021 study investigated the impact crises such as pandemics have in 20 United States cities with the highest incidence of people experiencing homelessness. They concluded that a combination of periods of high threat and high uncertainty disrupt a host of social and organizational processes.[19]

A 4-element model extrapolated from existing crisis response models shows 4 critical responses necessary for reducing the disruptions from a pandemic:[19]

1. Administration and leadership,
2. Continuity of services,
3. Financial resources,
4. Collaborations

SM and MM both serve essential roles in reducing disruptions during crises as it relates to this 4-element model. Even in non-pandemic settings, the CDC recognizes the importance of uninterrupted delivery of healthcare services for optimal population health. A framework stressed by the CDC focuses on 3 areas of disease prevention:[20]

1. Traditional clinical preventative interventions
2. Innovative preventive interventions that extend care outside of the clinical setting
3. Total community-wide interventions

SM and MM practitioners stand ready to respond to meet the demands of the future, pandemic or not.[19] This was demonstrated by SM programs rising to the occasion as the first line of defense at the height of the COVID-19 pandemic. As many non-medical outreach teams ceased outreach amid rising cases, the responsibility for crisis management was placed on SM teams. Qualitative reports demonstrate successful outcomes regarding screening, care, and containment of homeless populations, illustrating the value of SM/MM in crisis response.[21]

Benefits of Street Medicine and Mobile Medicine

As noted, MM and SM provide a crucial component of healthcare for at-risk populations. Target populations can include people experiencing homelessness, immigrants and migrant workers, runaways, and/or the underinsured and uninsured.[11] The success of both healthcare delivery models is secondary to flexibility, fostering trust, adaptation, and targeting the community's needs to create community-clinical linkages.[11,13] Opioid and substance use disorder, obesity management, and safe sex interventions are some examples of care delivered by MM and SM practitioners, with the successful outcomes at least partially attributed to the more tailored delivery method of these models.

In addition to bridging the gap often overlooked by traditional healthcare settings, innovative approaches to healthcare delivery, such as MM and SM, can help reduce patient reluctance to engage in healthcare by developing close personal relationships.[10] Meeting patients where they reside shifts the power dynamic in the patient's favor. It helps establish trust, especially for patients who have experienced negative encounters in traditional medical settings. This creates a sense of caring for the patient and can empower patients via a therapeutic alliance and patient agency to help mitigate unnecessary emergency department (ED) related costs while also freeing up resources for higher acuity patients.[11]

Offering care outside of fixed sites also provides the opportunity to extend essential veterinary services to homeless individuals' pets. It is estimated that 20% of those experiencing homelessness own pets, with growing evidence that pet ownership has been shown to positively influence the owners' sense of self-worth.[22] Street veterinary medicine not only promotes the well-being of the animals, but also further fosters trust between their owners, highlighting the importance of collaborative approaches in the care of people experiencing homelessness.

While formal data is limited, existing literature has demonstrated cost-effective outcomes of SM/MM programs by reducing avoidable ED and hospital utilization costs. The healthcare utilization expenses incurred by people experiencing homelessness currently are 5 times the national average.[23] This figure is even more impressive if looking at unsheltered adults specifically. A 2021 Boston Health Care for The Homeless Program study found that "unsheltered adults average $32,331 in healthcare spending per person per year." This amount is 3 to 4 times that of their sheltered homeless counterparts.[24] These high costs mainly stem from a disproportionate dependence on EDs for routine medical needs and increased hospital admissions rates due to advanced-stage illnesses.

SM and MM programs reduce healthcare misutilization and prevent costly complications by routinely treating acute illnesses and managing chronic diseases before they progress. An analysis by Lynch and colleagues in 2022 found that a theoretic 15% reduction in ED, hospital, and skilled nursing facility costs could generate over $9000 in savings per patient per year. This is more than enough to offset the average annual SM program cost of $3000-$9000 per patient.[17] One example of successful outcomes in practice is the Lehigh Valley Health Network (LVHN) SM program based in Allentown, Pennsylvania. In a span of 2 years, the program cut ED visits among participants by approximately 75% and reduced admissions by around 66%, resulting in $3.7 million in savings to the LVHN hospital network in fiscal year 2017.[25]

Novel approaches to healthcare delivery, such as SM and MM, can also help address both continuity of services and collaborations. These services provide greater accessibility to care without sacrificing quality.[11] In addition to people experiencing homelessness, other vulnerable populations, such as pediatric patients, are at an increased risk of experiencing barriers to accessing healthcare during pandemics such as COVID-19. The rate of pediatric preventative care and routine vaccinations decreased dramatically throughout the United States due to COVID-19.[18] Abigail Leibowitz of the Harvard Chan School of Public Health notes, *"Mobile health clinics are an underutilized, valuable method for delivering comprehensive, high-quality care to the most difficult-to-reach patient populations."*[18]

Economic Considerations of Street Medicine and Mobile Medicine

Despite the demonstrated potential for SM and MM programs to reduce overall per-patient costs, the steep startup costs of delivering this care remain a significant barrier. As reported by Mobile Health Map, a program run by Harvard Medical School that serves as the only comprehensive database of mobile clinics operating in the United States, the average annual cost of operating just one mobile clinic can exceed $630,000. For those clinics providing preventative and primary care, the average yearly cost balloons up to $980,000.[13] But who pays for these services? Of over 280 MHCs reporting to Mobile Health Map, 52% received funding from philanthropic sources, 45% received federal funding, 38% earned revenue from public insurance, and 37% received funding from private insurance.[13]

Billing to organizations (commercial insurance, Medicare, and/or Medicaid) is often a significant barrier due to issues with reduced billable visits, clerical costs, and administrative burdens. Funding for SM, in particular, has faced tremendous hurdles regarding reimbursement.[11] Despite many unsheltered people automatically qualifying for Medicare and Medicaid, SM providers often could not obtain reimbursement due to an issue with the *'Place of Service Code'* requirement and a bridge or tent is not a choice on the billing form. However, after years of advocacy from the SM community, as of June 23, 2023, a new *'Place of Service'* code was introduced for non-permanent locations, enabling SM to become reimbursable nationwide.[26]

MHCs serve as a service site for malpractice eligibility and claims submissions for commercial insurance, whereby SM practitioners are limited for billing claims as services rendered simply do not fit into a traditional clinical setting.[23] During the COVID-19 pandemic, temporary changes in telemedicine and MM regulations allowed for improvements to billing structures. Still, it is unclear if the federal government will revert those regulations in the coming future.[18]

Limitations of Street Medicine and Mobile Medicine

SM and MM initiatives face several limitations that hinder their effectiveness, including fragmentation of care, spatial and structural constraints, logistical challenges, and safety concerns.[11] Fragmentation of care is due to the inconsistent integration of SM and MM programs into mainstream healthcare systems, resulting in inadequate access to necessary specialists and follow-up services. Spatial and structural constraints include disruptions in privacy due to tight spaces within mobile units or on streets. This also refers to the limitations of medical equipment with SM practitioners often restricted to lower-quality portable screening tools.[27–29] Logistical challenges include the lack of suitable locations to park a vehicle for MM safely and safely storing and dispensing medication for SM.[2,11,30] In both programs, safety concerns are related to providing care in unpredictable and potentially hazardous environments.

Efforts are being made to improve modifiable limitations, especially fragmentation of care. The National Mobile Healthcare Association (NMHA) offers annual conferences, online resources, and regional coalitions to support existing and upcoming programs to better meet the needs of their patients. Additionally, NMHA offers Intensive Training Courses for both novice and experienced providers to disseminate frontline knowledge. The SM practitioners can often be siloed but the NHMA offers a community of like-minded practitioners. Their emphasis is on program sustainability, allowing the outreach to offer long-term support and continuity for patients. Often this starts with a needs assessment and a clear mission and can be facilitated by tools provided by the NMHA who supply comprehensive start-up checklists and peer support.

Next Steps and Future Considerations

Healthcare educators play a pivotal role in the future of SM and MM. It is hard for healthcare students to ignore specific social determinants of health when interacting with unhoused patients where they live and survive. While a small number of academic institutions are embracing SM, more work is needed if this movement is to be successful. Typically, these educational programs are pioneered by a passionate faculty member working with students to see patients outside the standard clinic setting.[4] As the focus shifts away from healthcare systems to more of a focus on health disparities and social determinants of health, it stands to reason that MM and SM concepts can be taught to healthcare practitioners early in their training. This type of learning can be transformational for healthcare students while also providing crucial and meaningful care to those most in need.[4]

Despite operationally being a distinct field of medicine since the early 1990s, SM is not formally taught in most healthcare programs. As the need for novel forms of healthcare delivery rises in light of current systemic shortcomings, the formal inclusion of SM into medical, PA, and nursing school curricula is a logical next step. The goal is to equip health professions students with the unique skills required for successful SM tailored to local cultural knowledge, harm reduction strategies, and reality-based care.[4]

A small number of academic institutions have taken concrete actions to address these limitations. The University of Pittsburgh Medical Center (UPMC) has developed an SM Fellowship under the direction of Dr James Withers for physicians who are graduates of Internal Medicine, Family Medicine, or Social Medicine residencies. These practitioners have a vested interest in becoming SM physicians. The UPMC program emphasizes the importance of coordinating care between Pittsburgh's unsheltered and the local hospital systems. Keck School of Medicine at the University of Southern California has created an interdisciplinary SM fellowship under the direction of Brett Feldman, MSPAS, PA-C. The Keck Fellowship provides robust training on workforce development, practitioner education, and training on various funding pathways.

Anna Buchanan and Ali Dewald, 2nd-year medical students at the George Washington University (GWU), are among those involving students in SM/MM outreach. As founders of the new student group DC Interdisciplinary Student Health Alliance, the duo are launching an educational component on care for people experiencing homelessness, to involve students from GWU's Schools of Medicine, Public Health, and Law. The goal is to prepare the next generation of professionals to collaborate across disciplines, advocate for policy changes, and design interventions that address the root causes of homelessness. This approach acknowledges that homelessness is not solely a medical concern but a complex issue intertwined with legal, social, economic, and public health aspects.

SUMMARY

The adage *"to cure sometimes, to relieve often, to comfort always"* has been used to describe the role of practitioners since the 1800s. However, mainstream medicine frequently falls short for underserved communities, especially people experiencing homelessness. SM and MM alike provide crucial healthcare services to these vulnerable populations through patient-centered preventative care, immunizations, and primary care.[11,13] There is growing evidence that both types of services (SM and MM) result in compelling cost savings while improving health outcomes for the medically underserved.[11,18] Ignoring the numerous benefits of these new models of care will result in a lack of equitable health services.[11]

While these healthcare models exhibit great potential, they face financial challenges and limitations. The significant startup costs of operating Mobile Health Clinics and SM programs hinder their widespread adoption, though new reimbursement codes for SM signify progress. Fragmentation of care, spatial constraints, logistical issues, and safety concerns pose operational challenges. Nonetheless, utilizing these novel forms of healthcare delivery has been shown to reduce the use of ED and hospitalizations among unhoused populations. This leads to an overall reduction in healthcare costs. However, more studies need to be conducted to further demonstrate the cost-effectiveness of such programs.[11,23]

The broader integration of SM and MM is more than just a cost issue; it fundamentally ties back to how we educate future medical professionals. Despite homeless individuals constituting at least 0.3% of the nation's population and presenting with unique considerations for healthcare delivery, formal instruction on their care remains notably absent within medical education.[31] By including components on homeless healthcare, including SM and MM novel delivery methods, into medical education, we equip future clinicians with the skills needed to compassionately address the multi-faceted challenges faced by this underserved population.

CLINICS CARE POINTS

- Street Medicine and Mobile Medicine modalities help address preventable morbidity and mortality in vulnerable populations such as the unhoused.
- Specialty point of care provided can include services such as dental services, mammography, and ophthalmology screenings.
- In addition to standard preventative and primary care services, Street and Mobile Medicine practitioners coordinate care such as social services, housing assistance, and harm reduction specialists.
- Providers must be aware of safety concerns related to Street and Mobile Medicine care delivery due to the unpredictable and potentially hazardous environment.

DISCLOSURE

The authors have nothing to disclose.

REFERENCES

1. Withers J. Street medicine: an example of reality-based health care. J Health Care Poor Underserved 2011;22(1):1–4.
2. Doohan NC, Mishori R. Street medicine: creating a "classroom without walls" for teaching population health. Med Sci Educ 2020;30(1):513–21.
3. Purkey E, MacKenzie M. Experience of healthcare among the homeless and vulnerably housed a qualitative study: opportunities for equity-oriented health care. Int J Equity Health 2019;18(1):101.
4. Withers J, Kohl D. Bringing health professions education to patients on the streets. AMA J Ethics 2021;23(11):E858–63.
5. Enich M, Tiderington E, Ure A. Street medicine: a scoping review of program elements. Int J Homelessness 2022;12:1–49.
6. Kao H, Conant R, Soriano T, et al. The past, present, and future of house calls. Clin Geriatr Med 2009;25(1):19–34.
7. Meyer BD, Wyse A, Corinth K. The size and Census coverage of the U.S. homeless population. J Urban Econ 2023;136:103559.
8. Tsai J, Wilson M. COVID-19: a potential public health problem for homeless populations. Lancet Public Health 2020;5(4):e186–7.
9. Frankeberger J, Gagnon K, Withers J, et al. Harm reduction principles in a street medicine program: a qualitative study. Cult Med Psychiatry 2022. https://doi.org/10.1007/s11013-022-09807-z.
10. Maxwell D, Thomas J, Plassmeyer M. The dynamics of providing street medicine to a geographically diverse homeless population in Hawaii. J Evid-Based Soc Work 2023;20(5):743–64.
11. Yu SWY, Hill C, Ricks ML, et al. The scope and impact of mobile health clinics in the United States: a literature review. Int J Equity Health 2017;16(1):178.

12. Feldman BJ, Kim JS, Mosqueda L, et al. From the hospital to the streets: bringing care to the unsheltered homeless in Los Angeles. Healthcare 2021;9(3):100557.

13. Malone NC, Williams MM, Smith Fawzi MC, et al. Mobile health clinics in the United States. Int J Equity Health 2020;19(1):40.

14. Urrea B, Misra S, Plante TB, et al. Mobile health initiatives to improve outcomes in primary prevention of cardiovascular disease. Curr Treat Options Cardiovasc Med 2015;17(12):59.

15. Snapshot. Available at: https://www.mobilehealthmap.org/find-clinics/. Accessed September 6, 2023.

16. Find mobile clinics - mobile health map. mobile health map at harvard medical school. Available at: https://www.mobilehealthmap.org/find-clinics/. Accessed September 6, 2023.

17. Lynch KA, Harris T, Jain SH, et al. The case for mobile "street medicine" for patients experiencing homelessness. J Gen Intern Med 2022;37(15):3999–4001.

18. Leibowitz A, Livaditis L, Daftary G, et al. Using mobile clinics to deliver care to difficult-to-reach populations: a COVID-19 practice we should keep. Prev Med Rep 2021;24:101551.

19. Jang HS, Shi Y, Keyes L, et al. Responding to the needs of the homeless in the COVID-19 pandemic: a review of initiatives in 20 major U.S. cities. Int J Public Adm 2021;44(11–12):1006–17.

20. Auerbach J. The 3 buckets of prevention. J Public Health Manag Pract JPHMP 2016;22(3):215–8.

21. Joshi S, Mann Y, Petersen A, et al. Providing preventative care during the SARS-CoV-2 pandemic: street medicine interventions amongst those experiencing unsheltered homelessness in the city of detroit. Open Forum Infect Dis 2022;9(Supplement_2):1193. https://doi.org/10.1093/ofid/ofac492.1193.

22. Geller J. Street medicine: caring for the pets of the homeless in. Journal of the American Veterinary Medical Association 2022;260(2). Published January 14, 2022, Available at: https://avmajournals.avma.org/view/journals/javma/260/2/javma.21.05.0249.xml?tab_body=pdf. Accessed September 10, 2023.

23. Walton R. Street Medicine or Mobile Medical Unit? Considerations for Expanding Medical Outreach - National Health Care for the Homeless Council. Published February 10, 2022. Available at: https://nhchc.org/street-medicine-or-mobile-medical-unit-considerations-for-expanding-medical-outreach/. Accessed August 10, 2023.

24. Koh KA, Racine M, Gaeta JM, et al. Health Care Spending And Use Among People Experiencing Unstable Housing In The Era Of Accountable Care Organizations. Health Aff 2020;39(2):214–23.

25. McGinley, Laurie. In the woods and the shadows, street medicine treats the nation's homeless - The Washington Post. Washington Post. Available at: https://www.washingtonpost.com/national/health-science/in-the-woods-and-the-shadows-street-medicine-treats-the-nations-homeless/2017/11/21/6ef037e8-ca54-11e7-b0cf-7689a9f2d84e_story.html Accessed August 14, 2023.

26. New POS Code for Street Medicine from CMS!. Available at: https://www.streetmedicine.org/index.php?option=com_dailyplanetblog&view=entry&year=2023&month=06&day=27&id=33:new-pos-code-for-street-medicine-from-cms-.

27. Guruge S, Hunter J, Barker K, et al. Immigrant women's experiences of receiving care in a mobile health clinic. J Adv Nurs 2010;66(2):350–9.

28. Carmack HJ. "What happens on the van, stays on the van": the (re)structuring of privacy and disclosure scripts on an Appalachian mobile health clinic. Qual Health Res 2010;20(10):1393–405.

29. Chen YR, Chang-Halpenny C, Kumarasamy NA, et al. Perspectives of mobile versus fixed mammography in santa clara county, california: a focus group study. Cureus 2016;8(2):e494.
30. Tito E. Street medicine: barrier considerations for healthcare providers in the U.S. Cureus 2023;15(5):e38761.
31. The 2022 Annual Homelessness Assessment Report (AHAR to Congress) Part 1: Point-In-Time Estimates of Homelessness, December 2022.

Venomous Exposures
Land, Sea, and Air

Caitlin Arnone, MPAS, PA-C, CRA[a],*, Kerri Jack, MHS, PA-C[b],
Janelle Bludorn, MS, PA-C[c]

KEYWORDS

- Snake bite • Spider bite • Jellyfish • Stingray • Hymenoptera • Assassin bug

KEY POINTS

- Systemic symptoms of snake and spider envenomation may be nonspecific but distinct dermatologic manifestations can be key to early diagnosis and treatment.
- Many marine envenomation symptoms improve from submersion of the affected area in hot water, which causes denaturing of the protein in the venom.
- Hornets, wasps, and bee envenomations cause the most animal-related deaths per year, which makes rapid treatment of allergic reactions essential.

INTRODUCTION

Venomous creatures may be encountered in a variety of environments across broad geographic distributions in the United States, including the land, sea, and air. Envenomation occurs when an animal actively delivers venom into an individual, usually via bite or sting. Venomous animal exposures result in more than 1 million emergency department visits annually.[1] Venom, the toxic substance that is injected during an envenomation encounter, is often composed of complex chemical components and may result in a myriad of local and systemic manifestations, some of which may result in a myriad of local and systemic manifestations, some of which may be life or limb threatening. This highlights the importance of clinicians' ability to recognize clinical features to identify various envenomation syndrome types, differentiate mild from severe presentations, and provide appropriate workup and management.

This article provides an overview of various venomous exposures of creatures living in the land, sea, or air—both common and novel—including envenomation syndrome clinical presentation, diagnostics, and management.

---

[a] Thermo Fisher Scientific, 929 North Front Street, Wilmington, NC 28401, USA; [b] Chatham University Master of PA Studies Program, Woodland Road, Pittsburgh, PA 15232, USA; [c] Department of Family Medicine and Community Health, Duke University School of Medicine, 800 South Duke Street, Durham, NC 27701, USA
* Corresponding author.
E-mail address: cait.m.wright@gmail.com

Physician Assist Clin 9 (2024) 187–199
https://doi.org/10.1016/j.cpha.2023.11.003
2405-7991/24/© 2023 Elsevier Inc. All rights reserved.
physicianassistant.theclinics.com

ENVENOMATIONS ON LAND
Snake Envenomation

Most snake envenomation in the United States is due to *Crotalidae* species, or crotalids, which include rattlesnakes, copperheads, and cottonmouths (water moccasins).[2] Colloquially referred to as "pit vipers" due to heat-seeking pits behind the nostrils, these snakes are characterized by their triangle-shaped heads, elliptical eyes, and long fangs.[3,4] Notably, patient description of the offending snake is often unreliable.[5] Rattlesnakes live in all US states except Alaska, Hawaii, and Maine, whereas cottonmouths are localized to the southeast, and copperheads in the southeast, Mid-Atlantic, and south-central United States.

Annually, there are approximately 5000 snakebites in the United States, a subset of these is venomous.[3,6,7] Men aged 20 to 40 years are the most common demographic to experience snake envenomation, usually at dawn and dusk during summer months when crotalids are most active.[6] Although copperhead bites are the most common, severe envenomation syndrome and mortality is more likely with rattlesnake bites.[3]

Local manifestations occur with nearly all snakebites, due to either the bite itself or envenomation. For crotalid bites, expect a 2-puncture fang mark wound, specific to crotalids with their venom-delivering fangs (**Fig 1**). About one-quarter of all crotalid bites are "dry bites" in which venom is not injected; in these instances, only bite effects are present, usually the characteristic 2-puncture wound.[6,9]

Local envenomation effects are due to the rapid absorption and slow elimination of enzymatic venom, which most commonly results in pain, erythema, edema, blistering, and/or ecchymosis.[3] These signs usually develop within 1 hour but may be delayed up to 8 hours. On assessment, the leading edge of local findings should be demarcated

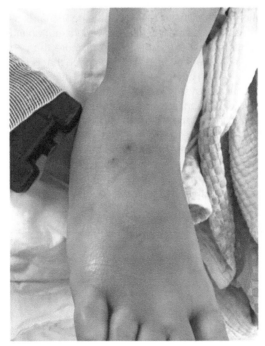

Fig. 1. Two-puncture fang mark of crotalid bite.[8] (Used with permission.)

(often with a marker) and reassessed every 15 to 30 minutes with inspection and palpation for proximal spread and progression to serious complications such as necrosis and compartment syndrome.

Systemic symptoms of crotalid envenomation include nausea, vomiting, paresthesia of the digits or perioral region, weakness, and myokymia, an involuntary fine rippling of muscles under the skin near the bite site or of the face. More ominous symptoms suggesting severe envenomation are tachycardia, tachypnea, hypotension, altered mental status, and coagulopathy.

Evaluation and management of any potentially venomous snakebite should prioritize assessment, stabilization, and periodic reassessment of airway, breathing, and circulation.[3] This may include managing shock with standard interventions or endotracheal intubation in the instance of bites to the neck and face, or angioedema.[3]

Initial laboratory studies for all bites should assess for hematotoxicity and rhabdomyolysis with the following:[7]

- Complete blood count
- Fibrinogen (if not available, D-Dimer may be obtained)
- Prothrombin time and international normalized ratio
- Partial thromboplastin time
- Comprehensive metabolic panel
- Creatine kinase
- Urinalysis

Electrocardiogram should be obtained for patients who have chest pain, dyspnea, or are critically ill.[7]

As venom-induced coagulopathy may be delayed, hematotoxicity laboratories should be repeated at 4 hours for all bites and continued to trend based on clinical status or normalization of laboratory values.

Management for all snakebites include stabilization of airway, breathing, and circulation, wound care, tetanus prophylaxis, analgesia, and consultation with Poison Control (1–800–222–1222, poison.org) or a medical toxicologist. Remove all jewelry and constrictive clothing and cleanse wounds, exploring and removing foreign bodies if present.[7] Relatively immobilize the affected limb, elevated to the level of the heart. Provide analgesia with acetaminophen and/or opioids; nonsteroidal anti-inflammatory drugs (NSAIDs) may be considered if the risk of coagulopathy/thrombocytopenia is deemed low.[7]

Administration of intravenous antivenom, under the guidance of Poison Control or a medical toxicologist, is indicated for envenomation associated with progressive edema, hematotoxcity, systemic symptoms, or bites to the face and neck. In the United States, there are 2 antivenom options: Crotalidae Polyvalent-immune Fab (Crofab, Conshohocken, PA, USA) and Crotalidae Immune F(ab')2 (AnaVip, Franklin, TN, USA) both with similar efficacy regardless of crotalid type.[10,11]

Snakes release the same amount of venom whether they are biting an adult or child, so antivenom doses are age and weight independent.[7] Crofab's loading dose is 4 to 6 vials.[10] If signs and symptoms progress, the loading dose may be repeated until control is achieved. Once progression halts, initiate a maintenance dose of 2 vials every 6 hours.[10] AnaVip's loading dose is 10 vials, which may be repeated if progression continues; there is no maintenance dosing recommendation.[11] Hypersensitivity is rare but serum sickness can occur in about a small percentage of patients who receive antivenom. All patients who require antivenom should be hospitalized for continued management and monitoring with serial examination and laboratory studies.

Spider Envenomation

The 2 venomous spiders in the United States are the black widow and the brown recluse. The former is found in all states but Alaska; the latter is concentrated in the southern Midwest and the South. Interestingly, most individuals who seek care for a chief concern of "spider bite" receive an ultimate diagnosis of dermatologic or soft tissue infection, not envenomation.[12]

Commonly encountered outdoors in landscaping or woodpiles, black widows have a characteristic red hourglass on the ventral abdomen.[13] Classically, their bite is painless and results in a target-appearing lesion with a central punctum atop a blanched patch surrounded by a ring of erythema.[14] Within a half hour to 2 hours after being bitten, individuals may develop systemic or musculoskeletal symptoms, indicative of moderate or severe envenomation. The local and systemic symptoms of black widow bites are termed latrodectism, which often includes myalgias, spasms, and rigid muscles of the limbs, abdomen, or back. Severe latrodectism may manifest with hypertension, tachypnea, gastrointestinal upset, and diaphoresis. At times, muscular rigidity and systemic symptoms may be so profound that they are mistaken for an acute surgical abdomen or myocardial infarction. Most latrodectism is self-limiting within 72 hours.[14]

Key components of black widow bite management include wound care, tetanus prophylaxis, and symptomatic management with medication such as analgesia for pain, antiemetics for nausea, and benzodiazepines for muscle spasm as needed.[15] For most patients, outpatient management is appropriate. Wounds should be cleaned with water and mild soap and then, to slow the spread of venom, cool packs may be applied while positioning the affected body part in a nondependent manner. For patients who exhibit latrodectism that is moderate or severe, Poison Control or medical toxicology should be consulted to guide administration of antivenom. Black widow antivenom is administered either intramuscularly or intravenously and may shorten the symptomatic period by 2 days and dampen severity of symptoms.[15] Because of the significant risk for this antivenom to result in adverse reactions including anaphylaxis, patients requiring this treatment should be closely monitored in the hospital.

Brown recluse spiders have a characteristic faint violin-shaped marking on their dorsum.[13] Exposure to these spiders typically occurs indoors in dark, isolated spaces such as closets or attics. Interestingly, they require counterpressure, such as putting a foot in a boot, in order to puncture human skin to cause a bite and/or envenomation. At the time of bite, an individual may note little to no pain, described as a burning sensation. Tiny puncture marks may be visible with or without associated erythema. However, because venom causes vasoconstriction during 2 to 8 hours, blanching with a raised rim of erythema develops with a crescendo of increased pain.[16] Most patients who experience brown recluse envenomation recover spontaneously; however, 1 in 10 cases do progress during the course of 1 to 5 days, manifested by tissue necrosis (**Fig. 2**). In this instance, hemorrhagic bullae develop at the bite site, evolving to eschar and ulceration with necrosis and granulation tissue.[16,17]

Rarely, within 1 to 2 days patients develop systemic symptoms: malaise, gastrointestinal upset, fever, myalgia, and/or dark urine. If present, these should raise suspicion for systemic toxicity prompting laboratory study workup for rare complications: hemolytic anemia, disseminated intravascular coagulation (DIC), or rhabdomyolysis.[18]

For brown recluse spider bites, management consists of wound care, analgesia, and tetanus prophylaxis. Similar to black widow envenomation local care, wash with gentle soap and water, apply cool packs, and maintain a nondependent position.[19] Debridement may be considered for patients who develop dermal necrosis

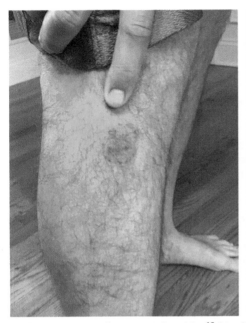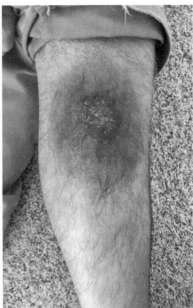

Fig. 2. Progression of Brown recluse bite.[16] (Used with permission.)

but it should be delayed until the lesion is clinically stable. Early debridement may lead to poorer healing and recurrent breakdown.[20] Dermal necrosis is amenable to treatment with antivenom; however, brown recluse antivenom is not available in the United States.

ENVENOMATION IN THE SEA
Jellyfish Envenomation

Jellyfish are found in all oceans but primarily inhabit shallow coastal waters. They are members of the phylum Cnidaria, and although there are 10,000 species of jellyfish, only 100 of these cause envenomation in humans.[21] Envenomation occurs when venom-containing cells (called cnidocytes) on tentacles are stimulated.[22]

The composition of jellyfish venom varies by species but can contain a variety of chemicals including catecholamines, histamines, lipases, and toxins. Cnidocytes are unique in that they can remain active for up to 2 weeks in tentacles that have broken off or on jellyfish that are dead.[21,23]

The venom released by cnidocytes can be toxic, although there are vastly differing degrees of toxicity depending on multiple factors, including the species as well as amount of venom injected.[22] Most lethal jellyfish reside in Australian waters, including the Australian Box Jellyfish and Irukandji box jellyfish, both of which can cause expeditious death secondary to cardiopulmonary effects.[22] The most common side effect of jellyfish stings encountered in the United States is localized pain, which can begin within minutes of making contact. This is often distributed linearly and can have an appearance similar to urticaria.[22]

Despite the common prevalence of jellyfish stings, there has been little evidence to suggest a preferred treatment.[24] It is well known that it is a priority to remove the clinging tentacles because there are still active cnidocytes that can continue to fire and release venom.[22]

Because of the differing composition of jellyfish venom, there is no universal treatment that applies to all stings. Pain management can be achieved with adequate analgesics and using hot/cold packs. Submerging the affected area in hot water (110°F–113°F) will help inactivate the proteins in the venom, thereby reducing pain.[22] Various topical recommendations have been explored including the application of vinegar, meat tenderizer, alcohol, and urine, although there are less data to recommend any one of these treatments.[24] It is recommended to rinse the affected area in salt water, not fresh water that encourages cnidocyte firing.[22]

In the rare event of contact with some of the more lethal jellyfish not local to the United States, treatment is supportive and may require medications to address side effects related to excessive catecholamine release. There is also an antivenom to the Australian Box Jellyfish, which has been known to cause death within minutes.[22]

Stingray Envenomation

Stingrays are flat, cartilaginous fish that can have very large wings reaching up to 3.6 m in diameter (**Fig. 3**).

Stingrays live in shallow water and like to hide under the sand. They do not actively seek out humans but when disturbed or threatened, will arc and thrash their barbed tail as a defense mechanism.[26] Because of this, injuries most commonly occur in the lower extremities. There are 2000 stingray injuries reported in the United States each year.[27]

The stingray causes its initial injury by the penetrating injury occurring from the serrated barb that enters the victim's skin. The barb is covered by a sheath, which on contact with a victim's skin, will break off and release toxins.[27]

A stingray injury causes immediate stabbing pain that can worsen for up to 2 hours after injury. Pain can spread across an entire limb and can cause associated erythema. Similar to jellyfish stings, the degree of pain experienced correlates to the amount of toxin released.[27]

The spine of the stingray is radiopaque, and because of this, x-ray is essential to evaluate the wound for barb location and/or retained foreign body after removal. In rare occasions, persistent wound problems can be caused by residual cartilaginous sheath within the wound, only identifiable by MRI.[28]

The venom itself is unstable and denatures when exposed to heat. Thus, similar to jellyfish stings, the best treatment is submersion of the affected area into hot water (max temperature of 113°F) for 30 to 90 minutes.[26,28]

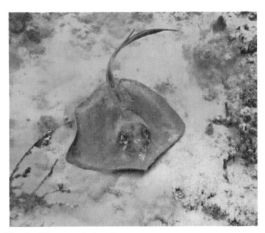

Fig. 3. Stingray.[25] (Used with permission.)

The stingray barb is serrated on both sides, with barbs directed the opposite way of tissue insertion, making removal very difficult.[28] A case report by Akar and colleagues[28] suggested a technique using 2 individuals, 2 surgical clamps, and a scalpel. They recommended linearly widening the incision 5 mm on either side of the wound to provide better access to the serrations. Using a clamp to stabilize the barb, a scalpel can be used to remove entangled tissues from the serrations on one side. An assistant then uses the clamp to hold open the wound to make sure that the tissues do not catch the spines of the barb while another person works on the other side.[28]

Once the barb and/or any broken fragments have been removed, the wound should be irrigated extensively, tetanus should be updated, and antimicrobial coverage should be given. A case study was done to evaluate what organisms would be of concern but little consistency was found.[29] Recommended antibiotics include ciprofloxacin, doxycycline, bactrim, and third-generation cephalosporins.[28,29]

Lionfish Envenomation

Lionfish are carnivorous fish native to the Indian and Pacific waters who are members of the scorpionfish family.[30] More than 30 years ago, they were introduced to Florida's coastal waters and have since become invasive to the southeastern United States. Because they feed on natural reef fish, their proliferation has caused a disruption to the ecosystem of coral reefs. Lionfish lack natural predators that would normally keep a species' population in check. This fact, combined with continually warming ocean temperatures, has led to their territorial expansion.[30,31]

Lionfish are unique fish due to their appearance; they are a beautiful brownish-maroon color lined with white stripes and have an eye-catching shape (**Fig 4**). In addition to tentacles above the mouth and eyes, they have stunning pectoral fins that fan out to the sides and 13 individual venomous dorsal spines, a combination that creates a dramatic appearance for snorkelers.[31]

The venom released by the spines that line a lionfish's body cause sensory and neuromuscular effects.[30] Individuals describe the associated pain as a "*searing, excruciating pain*" that can persist for up to several days. Similar to other marine envenomations, there can be associated erythema, swelling, and paresthesias.[30,31]

Treatment is aimed at controlling symptoms by submersion of the affected area in hot water (up to 110°F) for 30 to 90 minutes. This will improve pain by denaturing the protein in the venom.[30] Given the increased propensity to develop a secondary wound infection, it is recommended to treat these contact envenomations with oral doxycycline or a fluroquinolone, as well as updating an individual's tetanus vaccine if needed.[30]

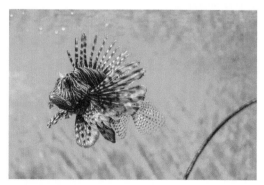

Fig. 4. Lionfish.[32] (Used with permission.)

ENVENOMATION IN THE AIR
Wasp and Bee Envenomation

Wasps and Bees are part of the Hymenoptera order of the family Apidae and Vespidae.[33] The Apidae family includes social honeybees, which can be found all over the United States, and African honeybees, which are found mostly in the Southwest United States, Florida, and South America.[34] The Vespidae family includes hornets, yellowjackets, and wasps, which are found in all 50 states.[33,34] Both inject venom through a modified ovipositor (stinger) in their abdomen. The sticker is a defense mechanism.[33] The difference between the 2 families is in the Apidae family the modified ovipositor has a barbed stinger that pulls the venom sac and stinger out. Thus, the stinger is used only once and stays in the victim. In the Vespidae family, the stinger is not barbed allowing for these insects to inflict multiple stings.[33]

Typically, the Apidae family is not aggressive and only sting when they feel threatened. The exception to this are Africanized honeybees, also known as "*killer bees*," which are very aggressive, defensive, and tend to swarm, leading to hundreds of stings.[33,34] The Vespidae family (wasps, hornets, and yellowjackets) tend to be more aggressive and territorial than bees and account for more stings due to their predatory tendencies.[33,35]

Hornets, wasps, and bees are the most common venomous animals, causing a majority of animal-related deaths, with an average of 72 deaths per year.[36] Honeybee venom allergies are the most common cause of anaphylaxis. This is thought to be due to the increase in frequency of attacks over time.[37] There are a higher number of sting-related deaths in men compared with women (84%) and within the age group 35 to 64 years.[38] There are certain occupations that have a higher risk of bee, wasp, and hornet stings: construction workers, landscapers, beekeepers, and exterminators.[33]

Hymenoptera venom is a complex mixture of allergic proteins, active antigens, peptides, amino acids, phospholipids, pheromones, volatile compounds predominated by water (>80%).[34,39] The protein mellitin is the main and most toxic component of bee venom, compromising 50% to 60% of the venom, and is the protein responsible for eliciting an allergic reaction and pain.[34] Wasp venom does not contain the protein mellitin but is composed of serotonin, wasp kinins, acetylcholine, and antigen 5, the main allergen in the venom.[34,35]

The usual reaction from a Hymenoptera sting is a local reaction (**Fig 5**) but some may develop an immunoglobulin E (IgE) immune-mediated allergic reaction, anaphylactic shock, or systemic toxic reactions.[34]

Those at highest risk of significant reactions from bee, wasp, or yellowjacket stings include those aged older than 60 years, small children, and those with other underlying comorbidities.[41] Hornet and bee envenomation reaction severity can also depend on the number of stings one sustains.[41]

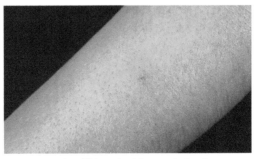

Fig. 5. Local reaction to wasp sting.[40] (Used with permission.)

Diagnosis is made based on history and physical examination findings. Individuals who have experienced systemic symptoms or a large local reaction (with a high risk of reenvenomation) should undergo allergy testing, although this testing is not recommended for screening purposes.[39] Allergy testing includes skin testing with venomous extracts, and should be performed within 2 weeks of the reaction to avoid false negatives.[39] Serologic testing for IgE antibodies or the use of component-resolved diagnostics, which tests for molecule-specific IgEs, can also be used.[39] If one is found to have IgE antibodies and has had systemic symptoms from a sting, venom immunotherapy can be given to reduce the risk of more severe reactions should one sustain future stings.[37,39] Treatment of Hymenoptera envenomation depends on the type of reaction (**Table 1**).[37,39,41]

ASSASSIN BUG ENVENOMATION

The Hemiptera order, commonly known as true bugs, include the Heteropteran subgroup, which is then further broken down into the Reduviidae family or assassin bugs.[42] Assassin bugs include several different species and all are venomous.[42]

Table 1
Response/symptoms to hymenoptera envenomation and treatment[37,39,41]

Severity	Type of Response	Symptom Timing	Signs + Symptoms	Treatment
Mild	Local reaction	Can last minutes to hours	• Pain • Erythema • Mild swelling	• Removal of stinger • Topical corticosteroids • Ice, tylenol, and NSAIDs
Moderate	Large local reaction	Can last up to a week	• Erythema >10 cm • Pain • Edema • Malaise • Fevers/chills • Headaches	• Removal of stinger • Oral corticosteroids • Oral antihistamines • Ice, tylenol, and NSAIDs
Severe	Anaphylactic response	Can occur within 10–15 min of sting	• Urticaria • Angioedema • Nausea • Vomiting • Hypotension • Dyspnea	• Removal of stinger • Epinephrine • Antihistamines • Cardiorespiratory support
Most severe	Toxic systemic reaction Serum sickness type	Can occur 2 d to 3 wk postenvenomation	• Vasculitis • Glomerulonephritis • DIC (disseminated intravascular coagulation) • Arthritis • Rhabdomyolysis • Hemolysis	• Removal of stinger • Epinephrine • Alkaline diuresis (*for severe rhabdomyolysis*) • Aggressive hydration • Dialysis • Cardiorespiratory support

Abbreviations: cm, centimeters; NSAIDS, nonsteroidal anti-inflammatory drugs.

They are characterized as predaceous: either hematophagous (blood feeding) or phytophagous (plant feeding). The broader category of true bugs are characterized by their unique elongated piercing, sucking mouthparts (proboscis), which is used for both feeding and injecting venom into its prey.[42,43] Assassin bugs are mostly found in the Southwest United States from Texas to California.

Predatory assassin bugs, including the ambush and wheel bug species, feed off insects but will bite humans when they feel threatened.[42] Their venom gland consists of 3 parts: the anterior main gland, the posterior main gland, and the accessory gland.[43,44] The anterior and posterior main glands secrete venoms made up of distinct proteins and peptides.[43] The venom from the posterior gland contains neurotoxins and causes immediate paralysis of the prey unlike the venom from the anterior gland, which causes no immediate harm.[43,44] In humans, the bite can cause a variety of symptoms ranging from pain, redness, swelling, and numbness (which can last several days) to tissue necrosis, respiratory symptoms, and very rarely death.[42,44]

Hematophagous assassin bugs include the *Kissing bug* species, which feeds on the blood of vertebrae. Kissing bugs are found in 27 states within the United States as far north as Pennsylvania.[45,46] They received their name due to their propensity to bite their victims on the mouth at night. These bites can cause an allergic reaction ranging from local symptoms of a papule or welt with a central punctum to an inflammatory infiltrate in the subcutaneous tissue to intense pruritus, pain, and lymphadenitis that can last up to 7 days.[46] These bites can also cause anaphylaxis with urticaria and angioedema.[41–43] Kissing bug venom is thought to inhibit voltage-gated sodium channels, which causes an anesthetic effect prohibiting humans from feeling the initial bite.[38] Kissing bugs are also known to spread the parasitic organism, *Trypanosoma cruzi*, which is found in their gastrointestinal system, causing Chagas disease.[46] Kissing bugs defecate on their prey when they are done feeding, which can cause *T cruzi* to be transferred when the host scratches or rubs the skin and the parasite then enters the wound.

Bites from assassin bugs are typically treated with oral antihistamines and analgesics after thorough cleaning of the bite with antiseptics. For anaphylaxis reactions, intravenous epinephrine is used as well as other supportive care. Patients with known reactions should carry an epi-pen especially if they are in endemic areas.[47]

Chagas disease is more common in Latin America but cases have been detected in the United States due to travels and Latin American immigrants.[45,46,48] Because of the risk of Chagas disease with kissing bugs, it is imperative that one seek medical attention if they believe they may have been bitten in order to obtain blood work for confirmation. During the acute phase, most are asymptomatic although they may develop the Romana sign (unilateral eyelid edema), malaise, fever, and/or lymphadenopathy. This acute phase can last 4 to 8 weeks.[46,48] Chronic infection occurs one to 2 months after initial infection. Approximately 30% to 40% of victims will develop a chronic infection along with major organ damage, usually cardiac.[48] Acute Chagas disease is treated with benznidazole and nifurtimox, the only 2 antitrypanosomal drugs available to treat acute infection. Chronic infection treatment with antitrypanosomal drugs is still under debate.[45,48]

SUMMARY

Venomous exposures can occur on land, in the sea, and in the air. Envenomation can occur from a bite, sting, through direct contact, or even a penetration injury. Initial local reactions are common with all envenomations and include pain, erythema, paresthesias, and edema. Although most envenomation injuries are not life threatening, clinicians should be familiar with the signs and symptoms of severe envenomation in order to efficiently diagnose and treat to prevent long-term complications.

CLINICS CARE POINTS

- IgE immune-mediated Hymenoptera venom allergy can lead to anaphylaxis and is imperative to diagnose in those who develop a large local reaction and systemic symptoms after a sting.
- Envenomation from true bug bites (assassin bugs and kissing bugs) typically induce only local reactions in humans, which are treated symptomatically but one must be aware of the possibility of Chagas disease with a kissing bug bite.
- About one-quarter of bites by venomous snakes are "dry bites" in which no venom is delivered.
- Black widow antivenom may result in severe allergy reaction or anaphylaxis. Brown recluse antivenom is not commercially available in the United States.
- Lionfish are an invasive species that due to their attractive appearance often attract snorkelers. Their venom causes localized discomfort.
- It is essential to make sure a stingray's barb is fully removed to avoid wound healing complications and infection.
- Most of the jellyfish in the United States coastal waters cause non–life-threatening stings that may be painful and cause other localized symptoms.

REFERENCES

1. Forrester JD, Forrester JD, Tennakoon L, et al. Mortality, hospital admission, and healthcare cost due to injury from venomous and non-venomous animal encounters in the USA: 5-year analysis of the National Emergency Department Sample. Trauma Surg Acute Care Open 2018. Available at: https://pubmed.ncbi.nlm.nih.gov/30623028/. Accessed August 23, 2023.
2. Venomous snakes. Centers for Disease Control and Prevention. Published June 28, 2021. Available at: https://www.cdc.gov/niosh/topics/snakes/default.html. Accessed August 23, 2023.
3. Warpinski GP, Ruha AM. North American envenomation syndromes. Emerg Med Clin North Am 2022;40(2):313–24.
4. Gold BS, Dart RC, Barish RA. Bites of venomous snakes. N Engl J Med 2002; 347(5):347–56.
5. Afroz A, Siddiquea BN, Shetty AN, et al. Assessing knowledge and awareness regarding snakebite and management of snakebite envenoming in healthcare workers and the general population: A systematic review and meta-analysis. PLoS Negl Trop Dis 2023;17(2):e0011048.
6. Buchanan JT, Thurman J. Crotalidae envenomation. In: StatPearls. ; 2023. Available at: http://www.ncbi.nlm.nih.gov/books/NBK551615/. Accessed August 23, 2023.
7. Ruha AM, Kleinschmidt KC, Greene S, et al. The epidemiology, clinical course, and management of snakebites in the North American snakebite registry. J Med Toxicol 2017;13(4):309–20.
8. Akoz A, Yildiz V, Orun S, et al. Management of Poisonous Snake Bites: Analysis of 29 Cases. J Clin Exp Investig 2018;9(4):140–4.

9. Kanaan NC, Ray J, Stewart M, et al. Wilderness Medical Society practice guidelines for the treatment of pitviper envenomations in the United States and Canada. Wilderness Environ Med 2015;26(4):472–87.

10. Dosing. CroFab 2023. Available at: https://crofab.com/treating-with-crofab/dosing. Accessed August 23, 2023.

11. ANAVIP® package Insert. ANAVIP® crotalidae immune F(ab')₂ (equine). Available at: https://anavip-us.com/pi/Accessed August 29, 2023.

12. Suchard JR. "Spider bite" lesions are usually diagnosed as skin and soft-tissue infections. J Emerg Med 2011;41(5):473–81.

13. Types of Venomous Spiders. Centers for Disease Control and Prevention. Available at: https://www.cdc.gov/niosh/topics/spiders/types.html. Accessed September 1, 2023.

14. Clark RF, Wethern-Kestner S, Vance M, et al. Clinical presentation and treatment of black widow spider envenomation: A review of 163 cases - ScienceDirect. Ann Emerg Med 1992;21(7):782–7.

15. Williams M, Anderson J, Nappe TM. Black widow spider toxicity. In: StatPearls. StatPearls Publishing; 2023. Available at: http://www.ncbi.nlm.nih.gov/books/NBK499987/. Accessed September 1, 2023.

16. Patti L, Bryczkowski C, Landgraf B. Brown Recluse Spider Bite. J Educ Teach Emerg Med 2019;30–2. https://doi.org/10.5070/M543044562.

17. Isbister GK, Fan HW. Spider bite. Lancet Lond Engl 2011;378(9808):2039–47.

18. Rosen JL, Dumitru JK, Langley EW, et al. Emergency department death from systemic loxoscelism. Ann Emerg Med 2012;60(4):439–41.

19. Anoka IA, Robb EL, Baker MB. Brown Recluse Spider Toxicity. In: StatPearls. StatPearls Publishing; 2023. Available at: http://www.ncbi.nlm.nih.gov/books/NBK537045/. Accessed September 1, 2023.

20. Nguyen N, Pandey M. Loxoscelism: Cutaneous and Hematologic Manifestations. Adv Hematol 2019;2019:4091278.

21. Cunha SA, Dinis-Oliveira RJ. Raising awareness on the clinical and forensic aspects of jellyfish stings: A worldwide increasing threat. Int J Environ Res Public Health 2022;19(14):8430.

22. DeLoughery EP. There's something in the water: An overview of jellyfish, their stings, and treatment. Int Marit Health 2022;73(4):199–202.

23. Jellyfish sting. Seattle Children's Hospital. Available at: https://www.seattlechildrens.org/conditions/a-z/jellyfish-sting/. Accessed August 3, 2023.

24. Ballesteros A, Marambio M, Fuentes V, et al. Differing effects of vinegar on pelagia noctiluca (Cnidaria: Scyphozoa) and carybdea marsupialis (Cnidaria: Cubozoa) stings—Implications for first aid protocols. Toxins 2021;13(8):509.

25. Green and black fish in body of water photo – Free St. john Image on Unsplash. Available at: https://unsplash.com/photos/cWu7zlPiorY. Accessed September 5, 2023.

26. Katzer RJ, Schultz C, Pham K, et al. The natural history of stingray injuries. Prehospital Disaster Med 2022;37(3):350–4.

27. Mora-Zamacona P, Águila-Ramírez RN, Muñoz-Ochoa M, et al. Stingray envenomation: Consequences of an embedded spine. Cureus 2023. https://doi.org/10.7759/cureus.38885.

28. Akar MS, Ulus SA, Durgut F, et al. A technical trick for extracting a stingray spine from hand: A case report. Acta Orthop Traumatol Turc 2022;56(5):347–9.

29. Cevik J, Hunter-Smith DJ, Rozen WM. Infections following stingray attacks: A case series and literature review of antimicrobial resistance and treatment. Travel Med Infect Dis 2022;47:102312.

30. Norton BB, Norton SA. Lionfish envenomation in Caribbean and Atlantic waters: Climate change and invasive species. Int J Womens Dermatol 2020;7(1):120–3.
31. US Department of Commerce NO and AA. What is a lionfish? National Oceanic and Atmospheric Administration. Published January 20, 2023. Available at: https://oceanservice.noaa.gov/facts/lionfish-facts.html. Accessed August 9, 2023.
32. Unsplash. Photo by Wai Siew on Unsplash. Published July 30, 2019. Accessed September 5, 2023. Available at: https://unsplash.com/photos/iFKMVFKY03c.
33. Arif F, Williams M. Hymenoptera stings. In: StatPearls. StatPearls Publishing; 2023. Available at: http://www.ncbi.nlm.nih.gov/books/NBK518972/. Accessed August 28, 2023.
34. Pucca MB, Cerni FA, Oliveira IS, et al. Bee updated: Current knowledge on bee venom and bee envenoming therapy. Front Immunol 2019;10:2090.
35. Fitzgerald KT, Flood AA. Hymenoptera stings. Clin Tech Small Anim Pract 2006; 21(4):194–204.
36. Xu Jiaquan. QuickStats: Number of deaths from hornet, wasp, and bee stings among males and females — National vital statistics System, United States, 2011–2021. MMWR. Morbidity and Mortality Weekly Report 2023. Available at: https://www.cdc.gov/mmwr/volumes/72/wr/mm7227a6.htm. Accessed August 28, 2023.
37. Burzyńska M, Piasecka-Kwiatkowska D. A review of honeybee venom allergens and allergenicity. Int J Mol Sci 2021;22(16):8371.
38. Forrester JA, Weiser TG, Forrester JD. An update on fatalities due to venomous and nonvenomous animals in the United States (2008–2015). Wilderness Environ Med 2018;29(1):36–44.
39. Matysiak J, Matuszewska E, Packi K, et al. Diagnosis of hymenoptera venom allergy: State of the art, challenges, and perspectives. Biomedicines 2022;10(9): 2170.
40. PHIL 21542. Public Health Image Library, Centers for Disease Control and Prevention; 1966. Available at: https://phil.cdc.gov/Details.aspx?pid=21543. Accessed September 5, 2023.
41. Schmidt JO. Clinical consequences of toxic envenomations by hymenoptera. Toxicon 2018;150:96–104.
42. Walker AA, Weirauch C, Fry BG, et al. Venoms of heteropteran insects: A treasure trove of diverse pharmacological toolkits. Toxins 2016;8(2):43.
43. Walker AA, Robinson SD, Yeates DK, et al. Entomo-venomics: The evolution, biology and biochemistry of insect venoms. Toxicon 2018;154:15–27.
44. Senji Laxme RR, Suranse V, Sunagar K. Arthropod venoms: Biochemistry, ecology and evolution. Toxicon 2019;158:84–103.
45. Bern C, Messenger L, Whitman J, et al. Chagas disease in the United States: A public health approach. Clin Microbiol Rev 2019;31(1):1–42.
46. Klotz SA, Dorn PL, Mosbacher M, et al. Kissing bugs in the United States: Risk for vector-borne disease in humans. Environ Health Insights 2014;8(Suppl 2):49–59.
47. Pereira Dos Santos CE, de Souza JR, Zanette RA, et al. Bite caused by the assassin bug zelus fabricius, 1803 (hemiptera; heteroptera: reduviidae) in a human. Wilderness Environ Med 2019;30(1):63–5.
48. Zemore ZM, Wills BK. Kissing bug bite. In: StatPearls. StatPearls Publishing; 2023. Available at: http://www.ncbi.nlm.nih.gov/books/NBK554472/. Accessed August 28, 2023.

Plants that Kill

Anna Mardis, PharmD Candidate 2024[a],
Darcie Evans, PharmD Candidate 2024[a],
Rebecca Maxson, PharmD, BCPS[a],*

KEYWORDS

- Toxic plants • Poisonous plants • Poison management

KEY POINTS

- Many commonly encountered plants have toxic effects on humans and animals.
- Toxicities can come from direct contact with or ingestion of plants.
- Toxic reactions may vary widely ranging from skin rash to death.

INTRODUCTION

In 2021, the National Poison Data System received 54,000 reports of possibly toxic plant exposures.[1] The severity of these exposures varies from simple skin reactions to death.[2] In 2017, Konstantatos and colleagues[3] reported a case where a male with prostate cancer in remission was found to have low pulse oximetry when he presented for a routine cystoscopy. Further investigation showed high levels of cyanide in his blood. The patient was self-prescribing ake (apricot kernel extract) for its purported anticancer properties. Many common fruits including apricots, peaches, pears, apples, and plums contain amygdalin in their leaves, bark, and seeds. When ingested, amygdalin is enzymatically converted to cyanide.[4]

Despite being "natural," several other plants can have toxic effects after contact or ingestion. In general, plant toxicity is not well studied when compared with toxicity from pharmaceuticals and risk is usually based on calls to poison control centers.[4] Standard treatment includes a period of observation to ensure serious symptoms are immediately managed with supportive treatment as needed.[4]

As identifying the plant exposure assists in diagnosis and treatment, the authors describe the typical reaction, type of exposure, and management strategies. Because the number of plants that may have some degree of toxic effect is far too numerous to be all inclusive, the authors have chosen plants based on the frequency of exposure and amount of available evidence and have organized them by human organ system. Plants are named based on their family (capitalized, plural, no italics), genus (capitalized, italics), and species (lowercase italics).[5]

---

[a] Auburn University Harrison College of Pharmacy, 1330 Walker Building, Auburn University, AL 36849, USA
* Corresponding author.
E-mail address: maxsora@auburn.edu

Physician Assist Clin 9 (2024) 201–216
https://doi.org/10.1016/j.cpha.2023.11.005
2405-7991/24/© 2023 Elsevier Inc. All rights reserved.

TOXIC PLANTS BY ORGAN SYSTEM
Skin

Skin toxicities by plants can be subdivided into irritant contact dermatitis (physical and/or chemical injury) which is most frequently seen and allergic dermatitis (immunologic response).[5]

Irritant contact dermatitis

Irritant contact dermatitis is caused when the skin comes into direct contact with the plant which can result in skin lesions, erythema, edema, pruritic papules, bullae, and ulcers which begin soon after exposure.[5,6]

- Stinging nettle (*Urtica dioica* L, **Fig. 1**) punctures the skin on contact, releasing an irritating sap, which usually results in a pruritic rash.[5]

- Buttercup (*Ranunculus* spp) species of plants contain an oil known as protoanemonin which is a direct irritant to the skin (**Fig. 2**).[5]

- Poinsettias (*Euphorbia pulcherrima*), a plant commonly seen around the winter holiday season, produces a milky latex on damage to the stems or leaves that is directly irritating to skin on contact.[6]

Treatment of irritant contact dermatitis is supportive in nature and may include over-the-counter anti-itch creams, topical or oral antihistamines, corticosteroid creams, and/or oral prednisone.[5,9]

Allergic contact dermatitis

Allergic contact dermatitis is caused when the skin is exposed to a plant containing oleoresins which trigger an immunologic response that may range from mild rash to immediate type 1 hypersensitivity reactions.[5,6]

- The Anacardiaceae species including plants commonly known as poison oak (*Toxicodendron diversilobum*), poison ivy (*Toxicodendron radicans*), and poison sumac (*Toxicodendron vernix*) contain urushiol compounds that trigger a delayed cell-mediated reaction involving T lymphocytes. Itching and redness occur 2 to 4 days after exposure unless the individual is previously sensitized in which case lesions can occur 8 hours after exposure.[5]
- Common ragweed (*Ambrosia artemisiifolia* L, **Fig. 3**) and other members of the Asteraceae species typically present as allergic rhinitis but may also cause an immediate type 1 hypersensitivity skin reaction.[5]

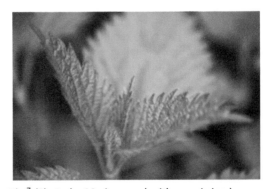

Fig. 1. Stinging nettle.[7] (Photo by Mariya; used with permission.)

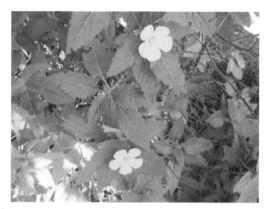

Fig. 2. Buttercup.[8] (Photo by Kim Zuber; used with permission.)

Treatment of allergic contact dermatitis is focused on symptomatic support and includes.

- Immediately rinsing (avoid scrubbing) the skin with soap and water
- Oral and/or topical steroids
- Cold water compresses or soaks three to four times daily which can include aluminum subacetate solutions (Burow's solution)
- Oral antihistamines for itching[5]

Gastrointestinal System

On ingestion, several plants can cause toxic gastrointestinal (GI) symptoms ranging from mild irritation to nausea and vomiting and even death.[6]

- Oxalate produced by dumb canes (*Dieffenbachia* spp) can cause oral mucosa irritation on ingestion. Management includes wiping the mouth with a cold wet cloth, washing the skin and eyes that came in contact with the plant and close monitoring of vital signs for symptomatic treatment (**Fig. 4**).[11]
- Holly (*Ilex aquifolium*) which is also more common during the winter holiday season can cause vomiting and diarrhea on ingestion (**Fig. 5**).[13]
- Buffalo beans (*Thermopsis rhombifolia*) have caused nausea, vomiting, dizziness, and abdominal discomfort in children. This plant has also caused death of livestock after ingestion.[6]

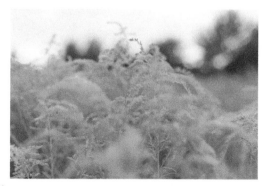

Fig. 3. Ragweed.[10] (Photo by Anastasia Lashkevich; used with permission.)

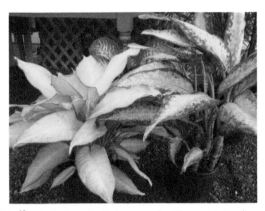

Fig. 4. Dieffenbachia.[12] (Photo by Kim Zuber; used with permission.)

- Pokeweed (*Phytolacca americana*), often used in the southern dish, poke salad, if not detoxified properly, can cause severe nausea and vomiting that has a foaming or soap-like consistency. Detoxification requires the leaves to be cooked by parboiling, which is when the plant is boiled twice and the water is changed between each boiling.[2,15]
- Death camas (*Toxicoscordion paniculatum*) results in milder symptoms of nausea, vomiting, and abdominal pain to more serious side effects such as bradycardia and hypotension when the bulb is ingested. Treatment is supportive and may include fluids and vasoconstrictive agents for hypotension as well as observation until vital signs normalize.[16]
- Castor beans (*Ricinus communis L*, **Fig. 6**) contain the toxin ricin. The largest concentration of ricin is found in the seeds and causes toxicity when the seeds are chewed and ingested. Symptoms occur within 24 hours of ingestion and may include gastroenteritis, nausea, vomiting, diarrhea, and abdominal pain. In severe cases, these symptoms may progress to hemorrhagic gastritis, hypovolemia, and hypotension. There is no antidote for this toxin.[17]

Cardiovascular System

Symptoms of cardiovascular toxicities include arrhythmias, hypotension, and, in some cases, sudden death.[4]

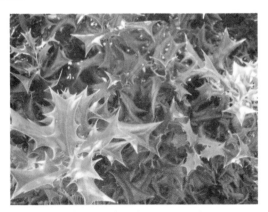

Fig. 5. Holly.[14] (Photo by Kim Zuber; used with permission.)

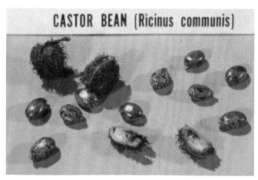

Fig. 6. Castor beans.[18] (Used with permission.)

- *Aconitum* plants including white monkshood (*Aconitum reclinatum*) and southern blue monkshood (*Aconitum uncinatum* L) produce alkaloids that can cause GI upset, central nervous system (CNS) effects, and/or irregular heartbeats and hypotension via slowing cardiac muscle repolarization. Ventricular arrhythmias are the most dangerous symptoms and require management with fluids, supplemental oxygen, and antiarrhythmic agents.[2,19]
- Mistletoe has been used in herbal medicine for centuries, but all parts of this plant can also be toxic when ingested in large amounts. American mistletoe (*Phoradendron flavescens*) produces phoratoxin that can cause hypotension, vasoconstriction, and bradycardia. Patients with dysrhythmias and electrolyte abnormalities should be hospitalized for observation and supportive care.[6,20]
- All parts of the English yew (*Taxus baccata*) contain taxine alkaloids. Eating a few yew berries is generally benign but GI distress can occur after 1 to 3 hours. Large ingestions can result in cardiac toxicity including all types of arrhythmias which can result in death. Of note, the chemotherapeutic agents, paclitaxel and docetaxel, were originally derived from yew bark (**Fig. 7**).[21]
- Oleander (*Nerium oleander*, **Fig. 8**) contains cardiac glycosides which are similar in structure to digitalis. Ingestion of flowers or chewing on leaves and stems first cause GI upset, but higher exposure can result in arrhythmias, hyperkalemia, and death. Case reports show that eating just 8 to 10 seeds can prove fatal to an adult. Treatment of poisoning is the same as for digitalis overdose.[2,6]
- Foxglove (*Digitalis purpurea*) flowers contain digitalis which can lead to GI symptoms and arrhythmias when ingested. Seeing yellow haloes is a classic symptom of foxglove poisoning and this reaction occurs with the pharmaceutical digoxin when at toxic levels.[24]

Liver

- Eating a wild mushroom commonly known as false morel (*Gyromitra esculenta*) can cause hepatitis induced by the toxin gyromitrin.[6]
- Death cap mushroom (*Amanita phalloides*, **Fig. 9**) is responsible for most fatal poisonings worldwide. It contains toxins that can inhibit protein synthesis leading to kidney and/or liver failure.[6]

Kidney and bladder

- The bracken fern (*Pteridium aquilinum*, **Fig. 10**) is a very commonly encountered plant that contains a carcinogen known to cause bladder cancer in animals as well as cancer of the mouth and throat in humans.[6]

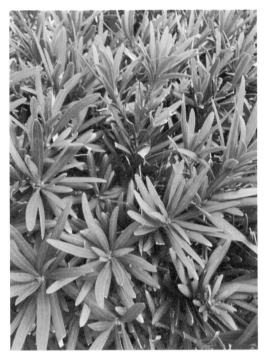

Fig. 7. English yew.[22] (Photo by Kim Zuber; used with permission.)

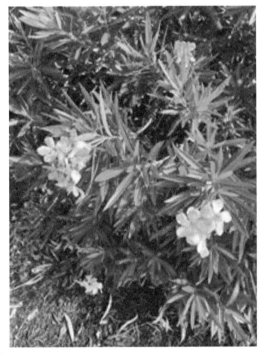

Fig. 8. Oleander.[23]. (Photo by Kim Zuber; used with permission.)

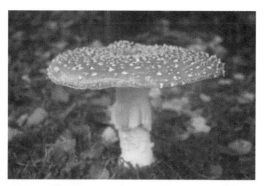

Fig. 9. Death cap mushroom.[25] (Photo by Guy Dwelly; used with permission.)

- Cortinarius species, which are a species of mushrooms, have been shown in clinical studies to cause acute kidney injury and death on ingestion. Deadly webcap (*Cortinarius rubellus*) contains a toxin orellanine that triggers kidney failure. Treatment includes supportive care, management of fluid and electrolyte balance, and the patient may require hemodialysis.[6]

Blood

- Fava beans (*Vicia faba*, **Fig. 11**) are generally benign unless ingested by someone with glucose-6-phosphate deficiency. For these individuals, ingesting fava beans can result in severe, life-threatening acute hemolytic anemia.[27]

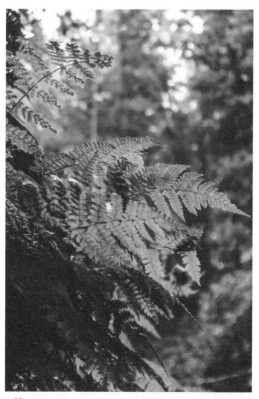

Fig. 10. Bracken fern.[26] (Photo by Aaron Buitenwerf; used with permission.)

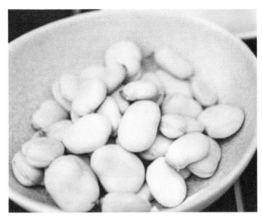

Fig. 11. Fava beans.[28] (Photo by Karolina Grabowska; used with permission.)

Nervous System

Symptoms associated with nervous system toxicities include dilated pupils, confusion, and paralysis. Paralysis of organ muscles can result in respiratory failure and incontinence. Paralysis of skeletal muscles is discussed in the skeletal muscle section.[4]

- Coniine, which is found in poison hemlock (*Conium maculatum*, **Fig. 12**), is an alkaloid that blocks nicotinic acetylcholine receptors which can result in GI upset

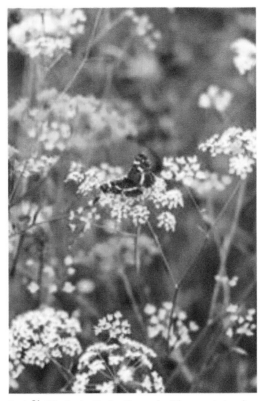

Fig. 12. Poison hemlock.[31] (Photo by Tudor S; used with permission.)

and muscle paralysis leading to respiratory failure and death. The philosopher Socrates was thought to be sentenced to death by poison hemlock.[29,30]

- Belladonna or nightshade (*Atropa belladonna*) causes delirium, hallucinations, dilated pupils, and rapid heartbeat on ingestion. All parts of the plant are toxic with the highest toxin concentration in roots and leaves followed by seeds and berries.[32]

Skeletal Muscle

- Buckthorn (*Karwinskia humboldtiana*) releases a neurotoxin that when chronically ingested can lead to paralysis which is often mistaken for Guillain-Barré syndrome. The highest concentration of toxin is found in the green fruit.[33]
- After ingestion of false lupine (*Thermopsis montana*), also known as mountain golden banner, livestock have been reported to experience locomotor depression and recumbency due to necrosis in skeletal muscle.[6]

IDENTIFICATION

Identifying the toxicologic etiology of a patient's symptoms may be difficult as there are so many possible options. To assist with this identification, **Table 1** lists the locations and physical features of the most frequently encountered toxic plants mentioned in this article. Gathering a detailed history from the patient and their care partners is key to properly identifying the offending agent and appropriately directing management.[4]

APPROACH TO MANAGING POISONOUS EXPOSURES

As clinicians, it is important to have a standard process to identify and manage patients presenting following a poisonous exposure. Guidance on how to triage patients with potential plant toxicities can be found in **Box 1** with details about Poison Control Centers found in **Box 2**. The clinical treatment goal is to allow for identification of toxicologic etiology and provide a more targeted management approach.[4]

Table 1 Identification for common plants (alphabetical by common name)		
Common Name (Scientific Name)	**Common Location**	**Physical Features**
American mistletoe (*P flavescens*)[20]	• Hemiparasite found on woody plants • Popular during holiday season indoors	• Shrubby stemmed plant (1–4 feet) • Light-green leaves • Small white berries in grape-like clusters
Belladonna or nightshade (*A belladonna*)[32]	• Ornamental plant	• Branching bush with oval leaves • Purple/black berries
Bracken fern (*P aquilinum*)[34]	• Moist open woodlands	• Branching black roots • Leaves arising from root up to 5 feet tall • Triangular-shaped leaves • Subleaflets are distinctly lobed at the base but not at the tip

(continued on next page)

Table 1
(continued)

Common Name (Scientific Name)	Common Location	Physical Features
Buckthorn (*K humboldtiana L*)[33]	• Semi-arid canyons and gullies in southwestern US	• Spineless, woody shrub (1–5 feet) • Clusters of green flowers product brown–black berries
Buffalo beans (*T rhombifolia*)[35]	• Dry prairies • Range lands	• Perennial (4–24 inches) • Yellow flowers • Blooms April to July
Buttercup (*Ranunculus* spp)[36]	• Ornamental plant • Generally wet areas	• Early spring bloomer • Perennial herbaceous plant • Yellow flowers
Castor beans (*R communis L*)[17]	• Moist, subtropical, and temperate climates • Disturbed soil	• Large shrub on woody stalks (4–5 feet) • Wide, green–red leaves • Brown/black spiny capsule fruit with gray/brown mottled seed
Deadly webcap mushroom (*C rubellus*)[37]	• Coniferous pine and spruce woods	• Grows August to November • Brown color • Radish like smell
Death camas (*T paniculatum*)[16]	• Low elevations • Moist, grassy meadows	• Perennial herb with tall, narrow leaves • Yellow or whitish green flowers in spring • "Onion-like" bulb without the smell
Death cap mushroom (*A phalloides*)[37]	• Broadleaved woods	• Tinted green cap, white stems and gills • Grows August to November
Dumb canes (*Dieffenbachia* spp)[11]	• High-humidity areas • Indoor potted plant	• Up to 6 feet • Broad, shiny leaves, variegated or spotted
English yew (*T baccata*)[21]	• Ornamental shrub	• Evergreen shrub • Glossy, dark green leaves spirally arrayed • Think bark that is red to red–brown and scaly
False lupine (*T montana*)[38]	• Well-drained soils of open woodlands • Great plants to intermountain regions	• Erect perennial (2 feet) • Yellow, pea-like flowers about an inch long
False morel (*G esculenta*)[39]	• Under pine trees	• Grows March to May • Red, brown cap on mushroom • Irregularly lobed with "brain like" cap appearance

(continued on next page)

Table 1 (*continued*)		
Common Name (Scientific Name)	**Common Location**	**Physical Features**
Foxglove (*D purpurea* L)[24]	• Ornamental plant	• Biennial herb • Simple, toothed leaves • Purple, pink, yellow or white tubular flowers on tall central stalk
Holly (*I aquifolium*)[13]	• Potted plant popular during holiday season • Moist, well-drained soils	• Deciduous and evergreen shrubs • Glossy green leaves, often prickly • Bright red berries
Oleander (*N oleander*)[40]	• Ornamental plant • Along highways • Potted house plant	• Evergreen shrub or small tree • Up to 25 feet tall • Narrow, sharply pointed leaves • White, pink, or red flowers • Fruit pods containing seeds
Poinsettias (*E pulcherrima*)[41]	• Potted houseplant popular during the holiday season • Tropics	• Large, green, bluntly toothed leaves and bracts (upper leaves) • Leaves change color from green to red in the blooming period
Poison hemlock (*C maculatum*)[30]	• Along roadsides • Ditches • Cultivated fields	• Biennial weed • Smooth branching stems with purple spots • Coarsely toothed leaves with fern like appearance • Strong pungent odor
Poison ivy (*T radicans*)[5,35]	• Pastures • Prairies • Woodlands • Rangelands	• Commonly a woody vine; small shrub in northern or western US • Multiple, small leaves arranged along stem
Poison oak (*T diversilobum*)[5]	• Eastern: Texas, northern Florida, New Jersey • Western: Pacific Coast from Mexico to Canada	• Eastern: erect, deciduous woody shrub • Western: woody, deciduous shrub (3–6 feet)
Poison sumac (*T vernix*)[5]	• Swamps and bogs in southeastern US	• Woody shrub or small tree • Seven to thirteen leaflet pairs per stem • Red fruit
Pokeweed (*P americana*)[15]	• Rich moist, open areas • Native weed, eastern US	• Large, perennial herb (3–10 feet tall) • Smooth, purple–green leaves • Clusters of berries (green when immature, dark purple when ripe)

(continued on next page)

Table 1
(continued)

Common Name (Scientific Name)	Common Location	Physical Features
Ragweed (*A artemisiifolia* L)[35]	• All types of soil • Disturbed places	• Annual (1–3 feet) • Flowers July to September • Simple green leaves (gray underneath) • Green–yellow male and female florets
Southern blue monkshood (*A uncinatum L*)[42]	• Low woods • Damp slopes • Along streams and in springs	• Resembles a vine • Several upward arching stems • Stems up to 5 feet long
Stinging nettle (*Urtica dioica L*)[35]	• Low, moist ground (ditches, open woodlands)	• Perennial (3–5 feet) • Thin dark green leaves with short stinging hairs • Flowers June to September • Green calyx without petals
White monkshood (*A reclinatum*)[42]	• Trailing along streams • In coves • Within mixed forests	• Up to 1 m tall perennial herb • Delicate stem • Flowers June to September

Abbreviations: Spp, species; L, Linnaeus; US, United States.

Box 1
Steps to assessing patient experiencing a potential poisoning[43,44]

1. Assess airway
   • Provide airway positioning

2. Assess breathing through oxygenation and ventilation
   • Provide supplemental oxygen and/or mechanical ventilation

3. Assess circulation and perfusion
   • Provide CPR, fluids, antiarrhythmics, and/or vasopressors

4. Assess CNS
   • Provide targeted therapy (such as benzodiazepines for seizure, cooling, and sedation for hyperthermia) as well as dextrose, naloxone, and/or thiamine as indicated.

5. Identify the toxin through history and physical examination
   • Discuss with poison control center
   • Treat the specific toxin (see **Box 2**)

6. Alter toxin pharmacokinetics
   • Decontamination, gastric emptying, and/or enhanced elimination through methods such as hemodialysis

7. Ongoing patient evaluation and treatment
   • ICU admission, psychiatric, and CV evaluation
   • Continued communication with poison control center

Abbreviations: CNS, central nervous system; CPR, cardiopulmonary resuscitation; CV, cardiovascular; ICU, intensive care unit.

> **Box 2**
> **Poison control center[45]**
>
> - If poisoning is suspected, contact the poison control center immediately.
> - Contact online at www.poison.org or phone at 1-800-222-1222.
> - Assistance is free.
> - Staffed 24 hours a day, 7 days a week, by specialists in poison information (primarily nurses or pharmacists).

SUMMARY

Although plants are typically seen as a harmless part of nature, they have risks of harm to humans and animals. It is important to be aware of the commonly encountered plants that have toxic potential and the effects of these toxicities which may occur through direct contact or ingestion. Treatment is directed toward the patient's symptoms and plant source. For some plants, all parts are poisonous, whereas for other plants, only certain parts maybe harmful. Clinicians should use a standard process to identify poisoned patients and provide treatment.

CLINICS CARE POINTS

> - Toxicities from plants happen from either direct contact or ingestion of the plant.
> - Reactions from toxic plants can affect many different organ systems and range from a simple skin rash to death, so it is important to take every exposure very seriously.
> - When assessing a patient with a suspected poisoning, assess their airway, circulation, and central nervous system first.
> - Collect a detailed history from the patient or their care partner to properly identify the toxicologic etiology and guide management.
> - The local poison control center is a valuable resource.
> - Frequent and prolonged monitoring of vital signs and symptoms may be necessary to ensure the safety of the patient.

DISCLOSURE

The authors declare no conflicts of interest.

REFERENCES

1. Gummin DD, Mowry JB, Beuhler MC, et al. 2021 annual report of the national poison data system (NPDS) from America's poison centers: 39th annual report. Coin Toxic 2022;60:1381–643.
2. Froberg B, Ibrahim D, Furbee RB. Plant poisoning. Emerg Med Clin North Am 2007;25(2):375–433.
3. Konstantatos A, Shiv Kumar M, Burrell A, et al. An unusual presentation of chronic cyanide toxicity from self-prescribed apricot kernel extract. BMJ Case Rep 2017. https://doi.org/10.1136/bcr-2017-220814. bcr-2017-220814.
4. Nelson L, Goldfrank LR. Chapter 118: Plants. In: Nelson L, Howland MA, Lewin NA, et al, editors. Goldfrank's toxicologic emergencies. 11th ed. McGraw

Hill; 2019. Available at: https://accesspharmacy.mhmedical.com/content.aspx?bookid=2569&sectionid=210276997. Accessed October 03, 2023.

5. Barceloux DG. Chapter 105: Plant dermatitis. In: Barceloux DG, editor. Medical toxicology of natural substances: foods, fungi, medicinal herbs, plants, and venomous animals. 1st ed. Hoboken: John Wiley and Sons, Inc; 2008. p. 677–89. Available at: https://onlinelibrary.wiley.com/doi/book/10.1002/9780470330319. Accessed October 03, 2023.

6. Watkins JB. Chapter 26: Toxic effects of plants and animals. In: Klaassen CD, editor. Casarett and doull's toxicology: the basic science of poisons. 9th ed. McGraw-Hill Education; 2019. Available at: https://accesspharmacy.mhmedical.com/content.aspx?bookid=2462&sectionid=202677479. Accessed October 03, 2023.

7. Mariya. Common Nettle Plant Macro Photography. Available at: https://www.pexels.com/photo/common-nettle-plant-macro-photography-11506323./. Accessed October 03, 2023.

8. Zuber K. Buttercup. 2023.

9. Cleveland Clinic. Contact dermatitis. Available at: https://my.clevelandclinic.org/health/diseases/6173-contact-dermatitis. Accessed October 03, 2023.

10. Lashkevich A. Yellow flowers of grass plants. Available at: https://www.pexels.com/photo/yellow-flowers-of-grass-plants-12477564/. Accessed October 11, 2023.

11. Barceloux DG. Chapter 125: Dieffenbachia and other oxalate-containing house plants. In: Barceloux DG, editor. Medical toxicology of natural substances: foods, fungi, medicinal herbs, plants, and venomous animals. 1st ed. Hoboken: John Wiley and Sons, Inc; 2008. p. 768–72. Available at: https://onlinelibrary.wiley.com/doi/book/10.1002/9780470330319. Accessed October 10, 2023.

12. Zuber K. Dieffenbachia. 2023.

13. Barceloux DG. Chapter 148: Holly (*Ilex* species). In: Barceloux DG, editor. Medical toxicology of natural substances: foods, fungi, medicinal herbs, plants, and venomous animals. 1st ed. Hoboken: John Wiley and Sons, Inc; 2008. p. 861–2. Available at: https://onlinelibrary.wiley.com/doi/book/10.1002/9780470330319. Accessed October 10, 2023.

14. Zuber K. Holly. 2023.

15. Barceloux DG. Chapter 132: Pokeweed (*Phytolacca americana* L.). In: Barceloux DG, editor. Medical toxicology of natural substances: foods, fungi, medicinal herbs, plants, and venomous animals. 1st ed. Hoboken: John Wiley and Sons, Inc; 2008. p. 800–2. Available at: https://onlinelibrary.wiley.com/doi/book/10.1002/9780470330319. Accessed October 10, 2023.

16. Barceloux DG. Chapter 109: Death camas. In: Barceloux DG, editor. Medical toxicology of natural substances: foods, fungi, medicinal herbs, plants, and venomous animals. 1st ed. Hoboken: John Wiley and Sons, Inc; 2008. p. 707–9. Available at: https://onlinelibrary.wiley.com/doi/book/10.1002/9780470330319. Accessed October 10, 2023.

17. Barceloux DG. Chapter 113: Castor bean and ricin (*Ricinus communis* L.). In: Barceloux DG, editor. Medical toxicology of natural substances: foods, fungi, medicinal herbs, plants, and venomous animals. 1st ed. Hoboken: John Wiley and Sons, Inc; 2008. p. 718–26. Available at: https://onlinelibrary.wiley.com/doi/book/10.1002/9780470330319. Accessed October 10, 2023.

18. PHIL 19559. Public Health Image Library, Centers for Disease Control and Prevention. Available at: https://phil.cdc.gov/Details.aspx?pid=19559. Accessed October 03, 2023.

19. Barceloux DG. Chapter 117: Aconite poisoning and monkshood. In: Barceloux DG, editor. Medical toxicology of natural substances: foods, fungi,

medicinal herbs, plants, and venomous animals. 1st ed. Hoboken: John Wiley and Sons, Inc; 2008. p. 736–42. Available at: https://onlinelibrary.wiley.com/doi/book/10.1002/9780470330319. Accessed October 10, 2023.

20. Barceloux DG. Chapter 130: Mistletoe. In: Barceloux DG, editor. Medical toxicology of natural substances: foods, fungi, medicinal herbs, plants, and venomous animals. 1st ed. Hoboken: John Wiley and Sons, Inc; 2008. p. 792–5. Available at: https://onlinelibrary.wiley.com/doi/book/10.1002/9780470330319. Accessed October 10, 2023.

21. Barceloux DG. Chapter 163: Yew (*Taxus* species). In: Barceloux DG, editor. Medical toxicology of natural substances: foods, fungi, medicinal herbs, plants, and venomous animals. 1st ed. Hoboken: John Wiley and Sons, Inc; 2008. p. 899–903. Available at: https://onlinelibrary.wiley.com/doi/book/10.1002/9780470330319. Accessed October 10, 2023.

22. Zuber K. English Yew. 2023.

23. Zuber K. Oleander. 2023.

24. Barceloux DG. Chapter 126: Digitalis-containing flowers. (foxglove, lily of the valley). In: Barceloux DG, editor. Medical toxicology of natural substances: foods, fungi, medicinal herbs, plants, and venomous animals. 1st ed. Hoboken: John Wiley and Sons, Inc; 2008. p. 773–5. Available at: https://onlinelibrary.wiley.com/doi/book/10.1002/9780470330319. Accessed October 10, 2023.

25. Dwelly G. Close-Up Shot of a Scarlet Death Cap Mushroom. Available at: https://www.pexels.com/photo/close-up-shot-of-a-scarlet-death-cap-mushroom-6418208/. Accessed October 03, 2023.

26. Buitenwerf A. Shallow Focus Photography of Green Ferns. Available at: https://www.pexels.com/photo/shallow-focus-photography-of-green-ferns-1293424/. Accessed October 03, 2023.

27. Luzzatto L, Arese P. Favism and glucose-6-phosphate dehydrogenase deficiency. N Engl J Med 2018;378:60–71.

28. Grabowska K. Fava Beans Green Ceramic Bowl. Available at: https://www.pexels.com/photo/fava-beans-green-ceramic-bowl-4963929/. Accessed October 03, 2023.

29. Hotti H, Rischer H. The killer of Socrates: coniine and related alkaloids in the plant kingdom. Molecules 2017;22:1962.

30. Barceloux DG. Chapter 131: Poison hemlock (*Conium maculatam* L.). In: Barceloux DG, editor. Medical toxicology of natural substances: foods, fungi, medicinal herbs, plants, and venomous animals. 1st ed. Hoboken: John Wiley and Sons, Inc; 2008. p. 796–9. Available at: https://onlinelibrary.wiley.com/doi/book/10.1002/9780470330319. Accessed October 10, 2023.

31. S T. Black and White Butterfly Perched on White Flower in Close Up Photography.; 2022. https://www.pexels.com/photo/field-flowers-summer-garden-13475029/. Accessed October 3, 2023.

32. Barceloux DG. Chapter 127: Jimson weed and other belladonna alkaloids. In: Barceloux DG, editor. Medical toxicology of natural substances: foods, fungi, medicinal herbs, plants, and venomous animals. 1st ed. Hoboken: John Wiley and Sons, Inc; 2008. p. 776–83. Available at: https://onlinelibrary.wiley.com/doi/book/10.1002/9780470330319. Accessed October 10, 2023.

33. Barceloux DG. Chapter 142: Buckthorn [*Karwinskia humboldtiana* (J.A. Schultes) Zucc.]. In: Barceloux DG, editor. Medical toxicology of natural substances: foods, fungi, medicinal herbs, plants, and venomous animals. 1st ediiton. Hoboken: John Wiley and Sons, Inc; 2008. p. 834–6. Available at: https://onlinelibrary.wiley.com/doi/book/10.1002/9780470330319. Accessed October 10, 2023.

34. Colorado State University. Guide to Poisonous Plants: Bracken fern, brake fern, eagle fern. Available at: https://poisonousplants.cvmbs.colostate.edu/Plants/Details/50. Accessed October 03, 2023.

35. Stubbendieck J, Carlson MP, Dunn CD, et al. Nebraska plants toxic to livestock: including bloat-causing plants rangeland, pastureland, and crop land. 2018. Available at: https://extensionpublications.unl.edu/assets/pdf/ec3037.pdf. Accessed October 11, 2023.

36. Colorado State University. Guide to Poisonous Plants: buttercup, crowsfoot. Available at: https://poisonousplants.cvmbs.colostate.edu/Plants/Details/88. Accessed October 11, 2023.

37. Keating H. Poisonous mushrooms: 8 most dangerous UK mushrooms. Available at: https://www.woodlandtrust.org.uk/blog/2022/10/poisonous-mushrooms/. Accessed October 11, 2023.

38. Colorado State University. Guide to Poisonous Plants: golden banner, yellow pea, false lupine. Available at: https://poisonousplants.cvmbs.colostate.edu/Plants/Details/19. Accessed October 11, 2023.

39. WildFoodUK. False Morel. Available at: https://www.wildfooduk.com/mushroom-guide/false-morel/. Accessed October 11, 2023.

40. Colorado State University. Guide to Poisonous Plants: Oleander, rose laurel. Available at: https://poisonousplants.cvmbs.colostate.edu/Plants/Details/60. Accessed October 03, 2023.

41. Colorado State University. Guide to Poisonous Plants: poinsettia. Available at: https://poisonousplants.cvmbs.colostate.edu/Plants/Details/115. Accessed October 11, 2023.

42. Colorado State University. Guide to Poisonous Plants: monkshood, aconite. Available at: https://poisonousplants.cvmbs.colostate.edu/Plants/Details/1. Accessed October 03, 2023.

43. Nelson LS, Howland M, Lewin NA, et al. Chapter 4: Principles of managing the acutely poisoned or overdosed patient. In: Nelson L, Howland MA, Lewin NA, et al, editors. Goldfrank's toxicologic emergencies. 11th ed. McGraw Hill; 2019. Available at: https://accesspharmacy.mhmedical.com/content.aspx?bookid=2569&sectionid=210267250. Accessed October 03, 2023.

44. Larsen LC, Cummings DM. Oral poisonings: guidelines for initial evaluation and treatment. Am Fam Physician 1998;57(1):85–92.

45. National Capital Poison Center. Poison Control. Available at: https://www.poison.org/. Accessed October 03, 2023.

Catching the Travel Bug
Travel Medicine in a Post-Pandemic World

John S. Lynch, DMSc, PA-C, DFAAPA

KEYWORDS

- Travel • Vaccines • Malaria • Yellow fever • Dengue

KEY POINTS

- Travel economics and travel medicine are innately inter-related.
- The importance of vaccines for travel cannot be understated.
- Travel medicine and the public health impact of diseases moving across borders is important to monitor.

INTRODUCTION

One significant driver of the United States economy is the travel and tourism industry. In 2019 it generated $1.9 trillion and brought nearly 80 million international travelers to the United States. This is in opposition to the $53.4 billion spent by US travelers abroad. Travelers contributed close to $240 billion dollars to the US economy in 2019.[1] Then, in 2020, the Covid-19 pandemic caused the travel and tourism industry to decline by 51%. International visitors to the United States in 2020 dropped by 76% with a slight rebound in 2021 (15%), more than the 2020 numbers. The travel/tourism industry further rebounded in 2022 with a 128% increase relative to 2021. This dramatic rise was likely a result of the United States easing COVID travel restrictions in November 2021.[2]

Travel data show a cyclical travel schedule with US citizens traveling mainly in July, June, and May. Foreign visitors to the United States peak in April, May, and July. Using data from 2017 (prior to the disruption that is Covid), females are more likely than males to travel (52 vs 44%), the average age was 44 for females and 46 for males, the average length of stay was 16.6 nights (consider incubation periods), and international travel destinations from the United States were dominated by the following countries:[3]

- Mexico
- Canada

Tidewater Physician Multispecialty Group (TPMG), Gastroenterology Williamsburg, 5424 Discovery Park Boulevard, Building B, Suite 104, Williamsburg, VA 23188, USA
E-mail address: cslasoz@aol.com

Physician Assist Clin 9 (2024) 217–228
https://doi.org/10.1016/j.cpha.2023.11.001
2405-7991/24/© 2023 Elsevier Inc. All rights reserved.

- United Kingdom
- Dominican Republic
- France
- Italy
- Germany
- Spain
- Jamaica
- China

For the reverse, foreigners coming to the United States, the statistics are slightly different. The top 10 countries sending visitors to the United States are as follows:

- United Kingdom
- South Korea
- Brazil
- Germany
- India
- France
- Japan
- Austria
- China
- Italy

The reason these data are important has to do with incubation periods, vectors, and exposures. All of these are important factors to look at when dealing with travel medicine.

Travel Medical Insurance

Based upon citizenship and availability of medical care, the cost of carrying medical insurance when traveling internationally is diverse among the many companies offering services. Benefits may vary widely. The Center for Disease Control and Prevention (CDC) puts out a Yellow Book offering details for the traveling public[4] (**Fig. 1**).

The 2024 edition of the yellow book, section 6, suggests links and information from multiple sources. As Medicare does not cover care outside the United States, '*Gap*' Policies are important. Medicare gap policies can cover emergency care but each policy needs to be reviewed closely. Our nephrology colleagues note that for '*dialysis cruises*', hemodialysis as covered by US insurance is only offered within 2 miles of US land (ie, the Virgin Islands, Puerto Rica, Alaska) and not on the cruise days that are outside of US waters. Many details can be ascertained from the state department info website: https://travel.state.gov/content/travel/en/international-travel/before-you-go/your-health-abroad/insurance-providers-overseas.html.

Five Travel Preparation Tips

Items that need to be considered as you embark on travel are the following.

- Vaccinations
- Prescription medications and legality in destination country
- Health insurance
- Copies of personal documents (ie, passport)
- An itinerary and contact information to nontraveling family/friends

Proper and timely vaccinations are effective means to prevent travel related illnesses above and beyond the usual childhood immunizations in the United States.

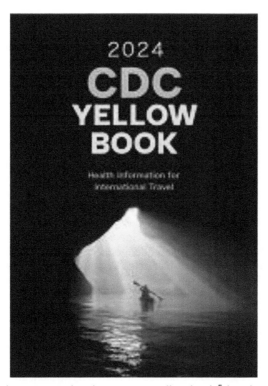

Fig. 1. Center for disease control and prevention yellow book.[5] (Used with permission.)

Travel vaccinations can include hepatitis A, rabies, typhoid, yellow fever, cholera, Japanese encephalitis, and tick-borne encephalitis. The CDC and the State Department websites are updated frequently for recommendations specific to country, area and type of terrain, and what you plan to do. Hiking through the Amazon requires significantly different vaccinations than a tour of South Korea.

Other Risks Associated with Travel

Jet lag
Jet lag can affect the most seasoned traveler. The general *'rule of thumb'* is that the number of time zones crossed equals number of symptomatic days. However, there are some ways to decrease the duration of jet lag. Sunlight and exercise help reduce to jet lag symptoms, and many travelers will change sleep patterns to mimic or approximate destination's time zone. Often a nighttime overseas flight with *'sleep'* (this can be tough) on the flight followed by staying awake all day as you arrive, might be helpful. Some sleep aides that are used include: zolpidem, triazolam, and/or melatonin. It helps to steer clear of alcohol, to stay hydrated, and to limit caffeine.[6]

Venous thromboembolism
Venous thromboembolism (VTE) is an umbrella term which includes deep veinous thrombosis (DVT) and pulmonary embolism (PE) The actual true incidence of DVT and PE related to prolonged air travel are low but are supported only by weak and variable clinical studies. Some studies suggest the incidence of symptomatic cases for VTE is 0.3% after travel of greater than 8 hours. There are risk factors that can increase

the chances of a DVT: obesity, past medical history of estrogen use, recent surgery. A *'soft'* risk pattern shows very short and very tall people at increased risk. That said, use of prophylactic anticoagulation is generally not recommended. There are suggested changes one can do while flying:[7,8]

- As window/middle seats may increase risks, select the aisle seats
- In-seat isometric calf muscle exercises
- Getting up and moving around
- Below the knee compression stockings

Diabetes and travel

Traveling for people with diabetes requires special consideration. It is not difficult to request a special meal and to pack diabetic injectable medication, medicine, and supplies in separate carry-on bag. The under-plane hold area may be too extreme for insulin. One can pre-arrange Transportation Security Administration (TSA) screening in the United States. This requires a call 72 hours prior to flying (TSA CARES 1–855–787–2227) to arrange for a *Passenger Support Specialist* to be at the checkpoint. It is suggested that you bring twice the anticipated medicine needed for the trip. Besides the TSA, the CDC and the American Diabetes Association (ADA) have excellent resources.[9–12] The ADA has a webpage devoted to diabetic supplies and air travel (https://diabetes.org/tools-support/know-your-rights/what-can-i-bring-with-me-on-plane).

Medications and travel

Medications available overseas often have different names. The classic example is acetaminophen, paracetamol internationally. Often planes use the international designation for medications so read the names carefully if using flight supplied medications on international flights. Pharmacy practices in each country are different, and you will need to research your destination prior to leaving the United States. Some medications that are over-the-counter (OTC) nationally are not internationally and vice versa. For example, birth control pills are OTC in Mexico and have been since the 1970s. Counterfeit medications can be an issue depending on travel site and a recent report of counterfeit medications sold at well-known pharmacies in Mexico has been reported by the Drug Enforcement Agency.[13]

Select Diseases

Malaria

Malaria is spread by the bite of the *Anopheles* mosquito with an incubation period of 9 to 18 days depending on the type of plasmodia (**Figs. 2** and **3**). As the average overseas trip is 16 days per the Department of Commerce statistics, there is ample time to develop malaria. Yet, one does not need to travel internationally to be exposed to malaria. There are multiple 2023 reports of in-situ transmission of malaria in Florida, Texas, and Maryland.[14]

If traveling to an endemic area, it is recommended that malaria prophylaxis medications be started. These include the following:[17]

- Artemether + lumefantrine
- Atovaquone
- Proguanil
- Chloroquine
- Doxycycline
- Hydroxychloroquine
- Mefloquine

MALARIA
Anopheles Mosquito

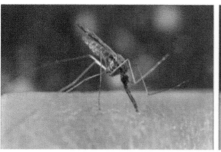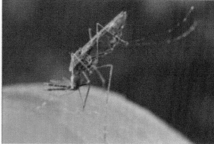

Fig. 2. Anopheles mosquito.[15] (Used with permission.)

- Primaquine
- Tafenoquine

There are multiple protocols depending on the where the traveler is going, underlying medical issues, and the resistance profile of travel. Be sure to check the CDC for updated information prior to traveling.

Prophylactic medications are often used for treatment when given in higher doses. These medications include the following:

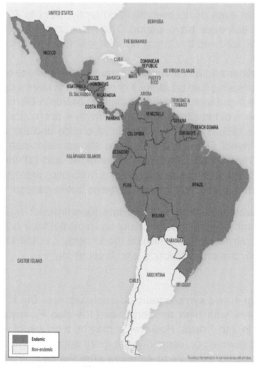

Fig. 3. 2021 distribution of malaria.[16] (Used with permission.)

- Artemether + lumefantrine
- Artesunate
- Chloroquine (a lot of resistance)
- Halofantrine
- Mefloquine (some resistance)
- Quinine
- TMP-SMX (lots of resistance)
- Tafenoquine (newest medication)

Terminal prophylaxis/treatment is either tafenoquine or primaquine. These are the only medications that can reach the malarial parasite while the parasite in sequestered in hepatocytes.[18] In pregnancy and breast feeding, recommendations may be different so be sure to check protocols. It is critical to determine the patient's G6PD status. If a patient is G6PD-deficient then they should not receive primaquine or tafenoquine as these medications may cause significant hemolysis. These two medications are not appropriate with pregnant patients or those breast-feeding children.[18]

Traveler's diarrhea

Traveler's diarrhea (TD) is one of the most common travel issues. While there are preventative protocols, bugs may overwhelm them:[19]

- Wash hands (clean water and soap, alcohol hand sanitizer)
- Be cautious with roadside food stands
- Eat thoroughly cooked meals
- Be cautious of bottled water in certain areas
- Boil, cook or peel foods as appropriate

It is estimated that even doing everything correctly, 30% to 70% of travelers will have diarrhea after a 2-week travel period. The most common bacterial infection is with *Escherichia coli*, followed by *Campylobacter jejuni*, *Shigella* spp., and *Salmonella* spp.[20]

The newest guidelines address severity and treatment. For those patients with mild to moderate cases, increasing fluid is helpful. For moderate to severe cases, bismuth subsalicylate, the active ingredient in adult formulations of Pepto-Bismol© will help. While there is some evidence of the effectiveness of bismuth + antibiotics, there has been an issue with antibiotic resistance. The antibiotic of choice and the use of prophylaxis guidelines have evolved. Fluroquinolones have shown resistance in *Campylobacter* and *Shigella* spp. There is also the issue of tendinitis and QT interval prolongation with fluroquinolones. For this reason, prophylaxis antibiotics are discouraged.

Treatment is guided by local resistance patterns but in general:[19,20]

- Mild TD: rehydration, bismuth subsalicylate, loperamide 2 mg 2-tab loading dose followed by 1 tab after each loose stool up to total 8 tabs in 24 hours
- Moderate TD: rehydration, loperamide monotherapy, antibiotic to be considered
- Severe TD: rehydration, antibiotics, and loperamide

Dengue fever

Dengue can present in two symptomatic characterizations: the first is a self-limiting disease that presents with high temperatures (104 deg F), myalgias, headaches, and rash that pass in 2 to 7 days. However, it may be a couple of weeks until the patients feels *'back to normal'*; or, secondly, the more aggressive form, *dengue hemorrhagic fever*, which can present 24 to 48 hours after the patient becomes afebrile. In this form, the patient develops abdominal pain, persistent vomiting, mucosal bleeding, edema, hepatomegaly, and/or a drop in hematocrit and platelets; all of which are very bad prognostic signs.

Dengue is another mosquito borne pathogen, passed by the *Aedes* species (*Ae. aegypti* or *Ae. albopictus*) mosquito. It is less common in the United States but there are pockets of dengue throughout the Americas (south and Central America) and throughout Equatorial Africa. Most cases seen in the United States are imported. Per CDC data, there were over 1200 cases in the United States in 2019.[21]

There is a quick and easy test for dengue called the '*tourniquet test*'. Take a patients' blood pressure with a sphygmomanometer in the biceps area. Calculate the middle of the systolic and diastolic readings and inflate the tourniquet to that. Leave on for 5 minutes and count petechiae in lower arm. If more than 10, this is a positive test (**Fig. 4**)[22]

Treatment is mainly symptomatic although fresh frozen plasma or blood transfusion may be needed in severe hemorrhagic dengue fever. There is a vaccine for dengue (Dengvaxia) but it is a live virus and care must be taken with immunocompromised patients.[23] Another issue is the cross reactivity of dengue and Covid. This can lead to false positive tests for dengue when patients actually had a recent Covid infection.[24]

Mpox

Mpox (formerly known as Monkeypox) is an orthopox virus passed via direct contact with contaminated surfaces. It will present with a rash that can be on the hands, feet, genitals, chest, etc. The rash looks like pimples or blisters and can go through several stages including scabs.[25,26] (**Fig. 5**) These lesions can be painful or itchy making diagnosis difficult. Incubation is between 3 to 17 days, and most people have no symptoms during the incubation time. Once the rash presents, patients can have symptoms including fever/chills, swollen lymph nodes, exhaustion, muscle aches and pains, or even respiratory symptoms. Treatment consists of symptomatic measures and use of certain antivirals under Food and Drug Administration (FDA) investigational new drug (IND) categorization. Brincidofovir is FDA approved for treatment of smallpox and other orthopox viruses; there is no data available concerning its effectiveness against Mpox virus. It is a prodrug for cidofovir which is used to treat cytomegalovirus. Cidofovir is an IND for use with Mpox as well. Combining brincidofovir with cidofovir when treating a patient is contraindicated.[27] A vaccine, Jynneos, is available for patients exposed to Mpoxor patients who are at high risk of contracting Mpox.[28] It is not considered a travel vaccine *per se*.

Mpox is the most recent example of the importance of the intersection between travel medicine and public health. As of 13 September, 2023, the CDC reported 89,889 Mpox cases worldwide (87,934 of them in areas without reports of historical Mpox) at 115

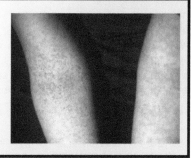

1. Take patient's blood pressure and record it.
2. Reinflate to midpoint reading between systolic and diastolic pressures (add the systolic and diastolic readings and divide by two).
3. Maintain midpoint reading for five minutes.
4. Deflate the cuff and wait two minutes.
5. Count petechiae below the antecubital fossa.

Positive test: ten-plus petechiae within a square inch.

https://www.cdc.gov/dengue/training/cme/ccm/tourniquet%20test_f.pdf

Fig. 4. Tourniquet test for dengue.[22] (Used with permission.)

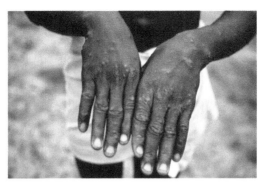

Fig. 5. Mpox.[26] (Used with permission.)

locations (108 of them without reports of historical Mpox).[29] Laos reported its very first case of Mpox on 20 September, 2023— a traveler from an adjacent country.[30]

Yellow fever

Yellow fever is another important disease at the public health-travel medicine interface. It is a fearsome disease, and few healthcare professionals in the United Status have seen a case of yellow fever. There is an effective vaccine against it which, in conjunction with mosquito control, banished yellow fever from the United States decades ago. Yellow fever vaccine is a mandatory vaccine for entry into many countries; the United States, however, does not require proof of yellow fever vaccination for entry. The CDC has a useful webpage providing country-specific data about yellow fever vaccination requirements and malaria prevention information:[31]

The disease's vector mosquito is present in the United States and is spreading. Its 2017 distribution is shown in **Fig. 6**.[32] There continue to be travelers from yellow fever endemic areas to the United States who may or may not have been immunized against yellow fever. Many of them arrive in Florida or New York.[33]

The yellow fever virus related to dengue virus, West Nile virus, Zika virus, hepatitis C virus, and others. It is endemic to large areas of sub-Saharan Africa and South America. Its' reservoir is jungle primates. There are 3 transmission cycles.

- Sylvan: jungle transmission, usually among apes but occasionally in humans working or living in the jungle
- Intermediate: a spill-over event from jungle transmission into towns and villages bordering the jungle
- Urban: propagation through humans in an urban setting

The latter is of the most concern.[34,35] It is estimated that over 200,000 people are infected annually with yellow fever, of whom more than 30,000 die.[34,36]

Yellow fever disease ranges from asymptomatic to severe hemorrhagic disease characterized by hepatitis and kidney failure. The jaundice and hematemesis associated with severe yellow fever cases earned it several nicknames: *Yellow Jack* or *the Black Vomit*. There is a 3–6-day incubation period followed by 3 distinct phases.

- Phase I is a short non-specific illness characterized by fever, headache, and malaise
- Phase II (or symptomatically frank yellow fever) presents with an abrupt onset of fever, chills, headache, low back pain, malaise, myalgia, nausea, dizziness, and Faget's sign (increased fever with decreased pulse)

CDC: Estimated Range of *Aedes aegypti* (2017)
Aedes aegypti mosquitoes

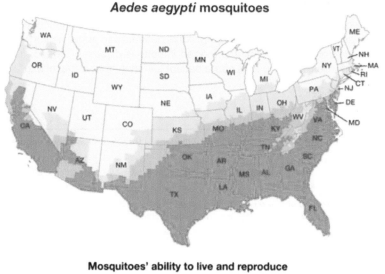

Mosquitoes' ability to live and reproduce

very unlikely   unlikely   likely   very likely

Fig. 6. Distribution of Aedes aegypti mosquitoes in the US. *Ae. aegypti*, also vectors, viruses responsible for dengue fever, West Nile fever, and Zika. (ESTIMATED potential range of Aedes aegypti and Aedes albopictus in the United States, 2017*. Retrieved from: https://www.cdc.gov/zika/pdfs/zika-mosquito-maps.pdf.)

- Phase III (or *"intoxication phase"*) can last 7 to 10 days and is characterized by the abrupt appearance of high fever, vomiting, epigastric pain, prostration, dehydration, petechiae, ecchymosis, epistaxis, gastrointestinal bleeding, hematemesis, and jaundice from severe liver and kidney damage.

Late neurologic symptoms such as confusion, seizures, and coma frequently presage death.[34,37] There is a fatality rate for severe disease of 20% to 60%.[38] Diagnosis is through blood screening and treatment is supportive.[34] Trials are underway with antiviral medications.[39–41]

SUMMARY

The general public seems to have caught a travel bug following the removal of Covid travel restrictions. International travel increased significantly between 2021 and 2022. International travel patterns to and from the United States seem to have changed, at least on the short term. A working knowledge of travel medicine and informational resources to help the traveler prepare for their journey will be much appreciated by the traveler. The knowledge will also be beneficial if the traveler catches a *bug* while overseas.

A change in frequency of travel from common points of origin of international travelers to the United States brings the threat of different diseases entities. South America has had intermittent outbreaks of yellow fever whereas Europe has not. There has not been a case of yellow fever in the United States for decades according to the CDC. However, yellow fever is a flavivirus transmitted by mosquitoes found in the United States, and the United States already has multiple other flaviviruses in the population: West Nile fever,

Zika, tick borne encephalitis, dengue. These diseases have been imported into the United States. Indeed, West Nile fever has established itself within our borders. The recent spread of Mpox (formerly known a monkey pox) around the world is certainly a travel-related disease. It has required extensive and expensive vaccination programs to control. Health care providers treating individual patients and public health agencies both play critical roles in combatting imported infectious diseases. Indeed, frontline practitioners may be the first to enounter a patient suffering from a "travel bug".

CLINICS CARE POINTS

- The dengue tourniquet test is easy to do and will identify those who have been exposed to dengue fever
- The importance of early vaccination during preparation for foreign travel is vital and should be reviewed with the patient
- During a history review one needs to look to travel to gauge the impact on both the health of the individual and for the community's public health at large

DISCLOSURE

The authors have nothing to disclose.

REFERENCES

1. National Travel and Tourism Office. International Visitation to and from the United States; Arrivals to the United States. Fact Sheet 2022. Available at: https://www.commerce.gov/news/fact-sheets/2022/06/fact-sheet-2022-national-travel-and-tourism-strategy, Accessed 26 September, 2023.
2. Department of Commerce; International Trade Administration. Interim study and report to Congress on the effects of the COVID-19 Pandemic on the travel and tourism industry of the United States. Available at: https://www.trade.gov/sites/default/files/2023-06/INTERIM%20REPORT%20TO%20CONGRESS%20-%20EFFECTS%20OF%20THE%20COVID19%20PANDEMIC_FINAL_0.pdf, Accessed 26 September, 2023.
3. Department of Commerce, International Trade Commission. Available at: Travel.-trade.gov/outreachpages/download_data_table/2017_Outbound_Analysis, Accessed 26 September, 2023.
4. Centers for Disease Control. Yellow Book 2024. Health Care Travel Abroad: Travel Insurance, Travel Health Insurance, and Medical Evacuation Insurance. Available at: https://www.nc.cdc.gov/travel/yellowbook/2024/health-care-abroad/insurance, Accessed 26 September, 2023.
5. Centers for Disease Control. Yellow Book 2004. Available at: https://www.nc.cdc.gov/travel/page/yellowbook-home, Accessed 26 September, 2023.
6. Goldstein CA. Jet Lag. (2023) Up-to Date. Available at:http://www.uptodate.com/contents/jet-lag?search=jet%20lag&sectionRank=2&usage_type=default&anchor=H3721224068&source=machineLearning&selectedTitle=1~22&display_rank=1#H3721224068, Accessed 26 September, 2023.
7. Douketis JD, Mithoowani S. Prevention of venous thromboembolism in adult travelers. (Aug 2023) Up-to-Date. Available at: https://www.uptodate.com/contents/prevention-of-venous-thromboembolism-in-adult-travelers?search=air%20travel

%20related%20DVT&source=search_result&selectedTitle=7~150&usage_
type=default&display_rank=7, Accessed 26 September, 2023.
8. Reyes N, Abe K. Deep vein thrombosis and pulmonary embolism. CDC Yellow Book; 2004. Available at: https://www.nc.cdc.gov/travel/yellowbook/2024/air-land-sea/deep-vein-thrombosis-and-pulmonary-embolism. Accessed 26 September, 2023.
9. TSA. Disabilities and Medical Conditions. Available at: https://www.tsa.gov/travel/special-procedures?field_disability_type=1008, Accessed 26 September, 2023.
10. TSA Insulin Supplies. Available at: https://www.tsa.gov/travel/security-screening/whatcanibring/items/insulin-supplies, Accessed 26 September, 2023.
11. CDC 21 Tips for Traveling with Diabetes. Available at: https://www.cdc.gov/diabetes/library/features/traveling-with-diabetes.html, Accessed 26 September, 2023.
12. American Diabetes Association. What can I bring with me on the plane. Available at: https://diabetes.org/tools-support/know-your-rights/what-can-i-bring-with-me-on-plane, Accessed 26 September, 2023.
13. U.S. Embassy Mexico. Health Alert: Counterfeit Pharmaceuticals, March 17, 2023. Available at: https://mx.usembassy.gov/health-alert-counterfiet-pharmaceuticals-march-172023/, Accessed 26 September, 2023.
14. CDC. Locally Acquired Cases of Malaria in Florida, Texas, and Maryland. Available at: https://www.cdc.gov/malaria/new_info/2023/malaria_florida, Accessed 26 September, 2023.
15. CDC Public Health Illustration Library. Anopheles Mosquitoes photograph identification numbers 18764 and 18763. Available at: https://phil.cdc.gov/Details.aspx?pid=18764 and https://phil.cdc.gov/Details.aspx?pid=18763, Accessed 26 September, 2023.
16. CDC Public Health Illustration Library. World wide distribution of malaria Available at: https://www.nc.cdc/travel/yellowbook/2018/infecious-diseases-related-to-travel/malaria5208 and https://wwwnc.cdc/travel/yellowbook/2018/infecious-diseases-related-to-travel/malaria5210, Accessed 26 September, 2023.
17. Tan KR. Prevention of malaria infection in travelers. Up-to-Date. Available at: https://www.uptodate.com/contents/prevention-of-malaria-infection-in-travelers?search=malaria%20treatment&source=search_result&selectedTitle=8~150&usage_type=default&display_rank=8, Accessed 26 September, 2023.
18. Centers for Disease Control. Treatment of Malaria Yellow Book 2024. Available at: https://www.nc.cdc.gov/travel/yellowbook/2024/infections-diseases/malaria#treatment, Accessed 26 September, 2023.
19. Riddle MS, Connor BA, Beeching NJ, et al. Guidelines for the prevention and treatment of travelers' diarrhea: a graded expert panel report. J Travel Med 2017 Apr 1;24(suppl_1):S57–74.
20. Centers for Disease Control. Travelers Diarrhea. Yellow Book 2024. Available at: https://www.nc.cdc.gov/travel/yellowbook/2024/preparing/travelers-diarrhea, Accessed 26 September, 2023.
21. Centers for Disease Control. Dengue. Available at: https://www.cdc.gov/dengue/, Accessed 26 September, 2023.
22. Centers for Disease Control. Tourniquet Test. Available at: https://www.cdc.gov/dengue/training/cme/ccm/tourniquet%20test_f.pdf, Accessed 26 September, 2023.
23. Federal Drug Administration DENGVAXIA insert. Available at: https://www.fda.gov/media/124379/download, Accessed 26 September, 2023.
24. Biswas S, Sukla S, Biswas S. COVID-19 virus infection and transmission are observably less in high dengue-endemic countries: Is preexposure to dengue

virus protective against COVID-19 severity and mortality? Will the reverser scenario be true? Clin Exp Investig 2020;1(2):1–5.

25. Centers for Disease Control. Mpox: clinical recognition. August 30, 2023. Available at: https://www.cdc.gov/poxvirus/mpox/clinicians/clinical-recognition.html, Accessed 26 September, 2023.

26. PHIL 12763 Characteristic mpox rash. https://phil.cdc.gov/Details.aspx?pid=12763, Accessed 26 September, 2023.

27. Centers for Disease Control. Mpox: clinical treatment; July 10, 2023. https://www.cdc.gov/poxvirus/mpox/clinicians/treatment.html, Accessed 26 September, 2023.

28. FDA. JYNNEOS insert. Available at: https://www.fda.gov/media/131078/. Accessed 26 September, 2023.

29. Centers for Disease Control. Mpox: 2022-2023 Global Map and Case Count. 13Sept2023. https://www.cdc.gov/poxvirus/mpox/response/2022/world-map.html, Accessed 26 September, 2023.

30. Promed. PRO/AH/EDR Mpox Update (40): worldwide, Congo DR, Laos. Archive number 20230926.8712311. Published Date: 26 September 2023. Available at: https://promedmail.org/promed-post/?id=8712311, Accessed 27 September, 2023.

31. Centers for Disease Control. Yellow fever vaccine and malaria prevention information, by country. Yellow Book, 2024. Available at: https://wwwnc.cdc.gov/travel/yellowbook/2024/preparing/yellow-fever-vaccine-malaria-prevention-by-country/, Accessed 27 September, 2023.

32. Distribution of Aedes aegypti mosquitoes in the United States, Centers for Disease Control Zika Virus webpage, https://www.cdc.gov/zika/vector/range.html, Accessed 13 July, 2020.

33. Dorigatti I, Morrison S, Donnelly CA, et al. Risk of yellow fever virus importation into the United States from Brazil, outbreak years 2016–2017 and 2017–2018. Sci Rep 2019;9:20420. https://doi.org/10.1038/s41598-019-56521-9.

34. Gardner CL, Ryman KD. Yellow fever: a reemerging threat. Clin Lab Med 2010;30(1):237–60.

35. Ndeffo-Mbah M, Pandey A. Global risk and elimination of yellow fever epidemics. J Inf Dis 2019;XX:1–9.

36. Centers for Disease Control. Yellow fever. Centers for Disease Control website, https://www.cdc.gov/globalhealth/newsroom/topics/yellowfever/index.html, Accessed 8 July, 2020.

37. Klitting R, Fischer C, Drexler JF, et al. What Does the Future Hold for Yellow Fever Virus? (II). Genes 2018;9(9):425.

38. Hamer DH, Angelo K, Caumes E, et al. Fatal yellow fever in travelers to Brazil, 2018. Morb Mortal Wkly Rep 2018;67:340–1.

39. Kleinert RDV, Montoya-Diaz E, Khera T, et al. Yellow fever: integrating current knowledge with technological innovations to identify strategies for controlling a re-emerging virus. Viruses 2019;11(10):960.

40. Gianchecchi E, Cianchi V, Torelli A, et al. Yellow Fever: Origin, Epidemiology, Preventive Strategies and Future Prospects. Vaccines (Basel) 2022 Feb 27;10(3):372.

41. Tomashek KM, Challberg M, Nayak SU, et al. Disease resurgence, production capability issues and safety concerns in the context of an aging population: is there a need for a new yellow fever vaccine? Vaccines 2019;7(179). https://doi.org/10.3390/vaccines7040179.

International Humanitarian Aid and Physician Assistants in Global Health

Mary Showstark, MPAS, PA-C[a],*, Mirela Bruza-Augatis, MS, PA-C[b]

KEYWORDS

- Humanitarian aid • Nonprofit • Physician assistant/physician associate
- Global health • Medical humanitarianism

KEY POINTS

- Learning the PA role in medical humanitarian aid.
- Preparing for international humanitarian aid travel.
- Working internationally with limited resources.

INTRODUCTION: MEDICAL HUMANITARIANISM AND GLOBAL HEALTH

International humanitarian organizations exist in many countries.[1] They are classified as intergovernmental organizations (IGOs) or nongovernmental organizations (NGOs). A treaty binds together an IGO that operates in more than one country and works toward a common goal or on issues of common interest.[2] These goals include addressing issues related to politics, culture, religion, trade, and health care. The United Nations (UN) and the World Health Organization (WHO) are examples of IGOs that participate in treaties.

NGOs generally do not involve the existing government and can work outside the government auspices. NGOs include nonprofit organizations (NPOs). NGOs may exist internationally, nationally, or at local levels. Some examples of health care NGOs/NPOs include Medicines Sans Frontiers (MSF, commonly known as *"Doctors without Borders"*), the Red Cross, and the International Medical Relief. The NPOs typically acquire their money through donations and grants.[3,4] A major funder for NGOs and governments alike is the World Bank. The World Bank's goal is a world free of poverty. The World Bank offers loans, credit lines, and grants to developing countries and is the largest funder of health care in impoverished regions.[5]

[a] Yale School of Medicine Physician Assistant Online Program, 100 Church Street South, Suite A230, New Haven, CT 06519, USA; [b] National Commission on Certification of Physician Assistants, 12000 Findley Road, Suite 100, Johns Creek, GA 30097, USA
* Corresponding author.
E-mail address: mary.showstark@yale.edu

Physician Assist Clin 9 (2024) 229–242
https://doi.org/10.1016/j.cpha.2023.08.006
2405-7991/24/© 2023 Elsevier Inc. All rights reserved.

NPOs, NGOs, and civil society organizations are terms that are often used interchangeably. On many occasions, IGOs and NGOs (including NPOs) collaborate for an intergovernmental/nongovernmental goal. Recent collaborations include the WHO declaring a Public Health Emergency of International Concern for the Ebola outbreak in Liberia and Sierra Leone in 2014. A similar situation occurred with the COVID-19 pandemic in 2020.[6] During health emergencies, many NPOs worked toward addressing the health care gaps in regional areas with the extra resources offered.

Some NGOs are already stationed in local areas and have extensive local knowledge of the people and their medical and cultural needs. Other NGOs rapidly mobilize to areas of concern. Emergency NGOs were among the first to arrive on Grand Bahama and the Abacos Islands in the Bahamas after Hurricane Dorian; in Beira, Mozambique, after Cyclone Ida; and in Louisiana, United States, after Hurricane Katrina. NGOs have assisted in natural disasters, including the earthquake in Nepal in 2015 and Haiti in 2010. Some NGOs work specifically in conflict zones such as Iraq, Yemen, South Sudan, and Cameroon.

Often each NGO may have different agenda and work in silos with little or no communication between other NGOs located in the same area. This lack of communication can lead to a duplication of efforts, supplies, and a lack of aid to the affected regions when more than one NGO sets up a health system. On the one hand, multiple NGOs help reduce patient load and have access to supplies and necessities such as clean water and support the local system. However, by creating a parallel health system, this can negatively impact the community. When a parallel health care system occurs, the local clinics and hospitals operate with lower treatment numbers, and a country often is unable to justify more health care workers. When NGOs leave an area, they may take the community facility where the locals were operating a clinic, leaving patients without access to care, medicines, or supplies. An example is Liberia, where there are 51 local doctors for 4.5 million people is presently the situation. This occurred because of an influx of temporary NGOs replacing the locally trained medical teams, who let all local physicians go and did not train new replacement doctors.

Thus, it is vital for medical humanitarian organizations to strengthen the local capacity in a region so a dearth of local providers will not be created when the NGO leaves.[7,8] The Paris Declaration on Aid Effectiveness and the Accra Agenda for Action asks for better communication and collaboration among NGOs. The goal is to create inclusive partnerships that achieve the end goal of better results and capacity development.[9] This would include standardizing measures of performance, simplifying donor procedures, and eliminating duplication of efforts. The WHO wants all teams responding to disasters to register with the WHO as Emergency Medical Teams (EMTs). The WHO has created standards for the EMTs and published them in the WHO *"Blue and Red Books."*[10] The Blue Book details the minimal standards required to become an EMT, and the Red Book details the engagement and management of EMTs and clinical response teams in armed conflict/complex emergency settings. However, many NGOs have yet to register with the WHO. Registration is rigorous with applications requiring teams to fill out paperwork, follow protocols, stockpile, and transport supplies to sites where they are needed. This can include a range of materials from tents to surgical equipment to medications.[10]

The UN and the WHO, as IGOs, have developed sustainable development goals. These goals were initially established in 2012 and updated for 2030. The 17 goals include disparate aims such as eradication of poverty and hunger, access to clean water, access to peace and gender equality, and climate change (**Fig. 1**).[11,12]

Many of the goals are influenced by social determinants of health (SDOH), which intersect with social and economic conditions in which people live, work, and access

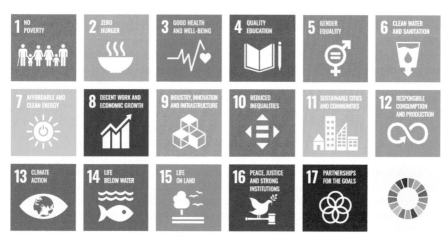

Fig. 1. The WHO sustainable goals.[13] (World Health Organization. Sustainable Development Goals. United Nations Foundation. Accessed August 16, 2020. The content of this publication has not been approved by the United Nations and does not reflect the views of the United Nations or its officials or Member States)

health care. SDOH includes financial stability, neighborhood and physical environment, education, food, community and social context, and health systems.[14,15] By highlighting these goals and SDOH, NGOs focus on how SDOH intersects with the medical care of patients. When COVID-19 (SARS-CoV-2) was first isolated, poorer outcomes occurred in patients with underlying conditions, including hypertension, diabetes, and obesity.[16] Limited access to food choices affects underlying health and leads to a higher likelihood of developing chronic disease (**Fig. 2**).

Economic Stability	Neighborhood and Physical Environment	Education	Food	Community and Social Context	Health Care System
Employment	Housing	Literacy	Hunger	Social integration	Health coverage
Income	Transportation	Language	Access to healthy options	Support systems	Provider availability
Expenses	Safety	Early childhood education		Community engagement	Provider linguistic and cultural competency
Debt	Parks	Vocational training		Discrimination	
Medical bills	Playgrounds				Quality of care
Support	Walkability	Higher education			

Health Outcomes
Mortality, Morbidity, Life Expectancy, Health Care Expenditures, Health Status, Functional Limitations

Fig. 2. Domains of social determination of health and health outcomes.[17] (Artiga S and Hinton E. Beyond Health Care: The Role of Social Determinants in Promoting Health and Health Equity. Kaiser Family Foundation. Published 2018. https://www.kff.org/racial-equity-and-health-policy/issue-brief/beyond-health-care-the-role-of-social-determinants-in-promoting-health-and-health-equity. Accessed August 20, 2023)

As a health care provider, one must identify and thoroughly research the international humanitarian aid organization one plans to participate with and be cognizant of the organization's reputation and footprint. Outside of global disasters, there is no centralized registry to report where NGOs are working, making this step a bit more challenging. The health care provider should attend a local or virtual meeting and meet members of the NGO team. Understanding how the organization is run, who is in charge, how communications work, who you are working with, and what your role will be is crucial. Will you have a full medical team, medications, medical equipment, and an interprofessional team with you? Will you be the only provider? How will you care for the patient, and in what capacity (field, make-shift hospital)? Who will help if something goes wrong (other trained providers, evacuation staff)? Will you be safe (especially important in conflict zones) and have access to personal protective equipment (PPE)? What is your role (medical treatment or building a hospital)? Then, there are the questions you need to ask yourself. Are you comfortable if you are not functioning in your usual role? How will you cope, work with limited resources and adjust to and respect cultural and religious differences? This article aims to walk the health care provider through these questions and how to get involved (**Table 1**).

Preplanning

Working with an NGO can be a rewarding experience. As many medical humanitarian organizations have varying financial and ancillary support staff levels, one cannot rely on an organization to do all the planning. You will need to take personal accountability for understanding where you will be and what you will need for your trip. Depending on your country of origin, locate the nearest consulate in the volunteer country in case of an emergency, disaster, or loss of passport/ID cards. You will also need to think about logistics. Do you have a passport/time to process a passport and a visa (if needed)? How will you get money, and will it be in the local currency? Should you go to a bank before your trip or on arrival? Does the country have the infrastructure (automatic teller

Table 1 How to get involved	
Steps	**Example**
Pick an organization you are passionate about	• Search NGO databases • PA for Global health Web site (www.pasforglobalhealth.com) • Review the mission statement and the objectives of the organization chosen
Research the organization	• Look at online reviews including charity ranking sites • GuideStar (https://www.guidestar.org/): connects donors to NGOs • Charity navigator (https://www.charitynavigator.org/): US-specific charity watchdog • Charity watch (https://www.charitywatch.org/): US-specific charity watchdog with contact between volunteers, sites
Attend a local or virtual meeting	• Monitor internal and external communication styles • Meet members of the team
Find a "good fit"	• What would be your role? • Medical or physical labor (IE: building hospital or clinic) • Will you be comfortable if you are not working in your role the whole time? • Who are the other members of your team?

machines [ATMs]) with the ability to withdraw money, or has the country just sustained a disaster or is in a conflict zone? Will you be going to multiple countries and need more than one currency? Some countries may only accept money in US dollars from all foreigners, no matter their country of origin. Therefore, locating nearby hospitals and pharmacies in case of an emergency and packing your personal items is essential. We suggest the following (**Tables 2** and **3**):

Table 2 Personal packing[18]	
Personal packing	**Examples**
Documents	• Copies of medical and driver's licenses • Passport and copies of passport and extra passport photos • Copies of travel visa (if applicable) • Copies of your itinerary • International health care insurance • Travel insurance/evacuation • Proof of vaccinations (PRN) • Copies of prescriptions (including generic names) • Emergency contact card: family, phone numbers, embassy, consulate information, and email addresses
Personal Care	• Hand sanitizer • Toilet paper/baby wipes • Laundry detergent, deodorant, soap, shampoo, toothpaste, toothbrush, dental floss, face cleanser, brush/comb, shaving cream, and supplies • Water purification tablets/SteriPen water purifier/water filtration system • Feminine-hygiene products (tampons), condoms/birth control methods • Nail file/clipper • Tweezers • Glasses/contacts (contact solution) • Medication/prescription (RX + OTC) • Medical alert bracelets (PRN)
Environmental Safety	• Appropriate clothing for the countries you are traveling to • Sunscreen with UVA/UVB protection • Sunglasses • Hat • Work gloves (leather or rubber) • Safety goggles • Flashlight/headlamp (include spare batteries) • Matches/lighter • Insect prevention (bed net and repellents) • Snacks/food • PPE
Other	• Earplugs, eye mask/bandana • Cell phone/electronics chargers (+ travel adapters, converters) • Ziploc bags • Credit/ATM cards/cash • Beacon • Travel backpack • Maps/guidebooks • Translation dictionary or offline language application

Abbreviations: ATM, automatic teller machine; OTC, over the counter; PPE, personal protective equipment; PRN, as needed; RX, prescription; UVA/UVB, ultraviolet light A/B.

Adapted from CDC. Pack Smart. Travelers' Health. Published 2019. Accessed July 31, 2020. https://wwwnc.cdc.gov/travel/page/pack-smart

Table 3	
Personal medical supplies for treating patients	
Personal medical supplies	• Stethoscope
	• Disposable gloves
	• Pulse oximeter
	• Thermometer
	• Blood pressure cuff
	• Flashlight
	• Trauma SHEARS (packed in luggage)
	• Scrubs
	• PPE (surgical and N95 masks, gowns, face shield)
	• Eye/ear protection (goggles, earplugs)
	• Notepad/pens (stickers if seeing children)
	• Pocket reference books/Pharmacopeia:

Note: Different names of medications exist for each country and the antibiotic resistance profile of each area is different (authors suggestions).

Personal Medications

Moreover, personal medications are essential for your safety. Some organizations may bring medicines with them; however, these medications are dedicated to the patients you will be managing and you should not rely on them. Thus, it is strongly recommended that you bring your own medications. For personal medicines, ensure that all medications are labeled with the prescription name and your name. You cannot rely on finding your medications abroad. Travel vaccines and prophylaxis medications should be purchased ahead of time. The International Society of Travel Medicine has listings of international clinics.[19]

The following medications are suggestions for personal care and safety (**Table 4**).

Medical Equipment and Medications

Medications and durable medical equipment (DME) may be needed on an international humanitarian aid trip. Some groups will supply this, whereas others will ask you to bring the DME. You cannot assume that DME is allowed into the country. You need to check with the organization first, their country's contact, the Ministry of Health, or the country's local consulate.

Table 4		
Medication suggestions for personal care and safety		
• First-Aid Kit (Mini)	• Over the counter pain meds	• Malaria prophylaxis (as indicated and prescribed)
• Personal prescriptions, original bottles with your name	• Over the counter laxative	• Antibiotics (in needed/as prescribed and directed)
• Antidiarrheals	• Sedative/sleep aid	• Rehydration salts
• Antihistamine	• Over the counter saline nose spray	• Gauze/bandages
• Motion sickness medication	• 1% Hydrocortisone cream (over the counter)	• Antifungal ointments
• Cough drops	• Antiseptic	• Antibacterial ointments
• Decongestant		
• Eye drops (as indicated and/or prescribed)		

Adapted from CDC. Traveling Abroad with Medicine. Traveler's Health. Published 2022. Accessed August 25, 2023. https://wwwnc.cdc.gov/travel/page/travel-abroad-with-medicine

The WHO has guidelines on bringing durable medical supplies. Donations should always benefit the end-user, that is, do not bring in a defibrillator without a plan to train the user on how to use the device. All equipment should be respectful and comply with government policies and regulations. Donations should have an intended recipient.[20,21] In Haiti, after the 2010 earthquake, many donations were left without recipients. The equipment sat on the side of the tarmac at the Port Au Prince airport and was subject to weather and looting. Generally, equipment will also need a plan for maintenance and calibration of goods. For instance, automatic external defibrillator pads expire, and iSTAT portable blood laboratory machines need regular calibration. Each piece of equipment needs a plan for maintenance. When working with an organization, a provider must aim to adhere to the WHO policies and uphold ethical standards when it comes to donations of medical supplies.[21]

Many organizations will bring medications and supplies to distribute to patients. Providers must note that expired medicines should not be donated, and the shelf life should be assessed before accepting these products.[20] Before one even attempts to bring medicine into a country, check to see if the medication is allowed. Some medications are legal in one country and illegal in others; for instance, in Japan, some allergy and sinus medications are forbidden.[22] You may be unable to clear customs if some medicines are found in your possession or if you carry an excessive supply. In the worst-case scenario, you may face imprisonment or even a death sentence.[23] The WHO also has guidelines on medication donations to assist the health care provider.[21]

If you are being asked by an NGO to bring certain medications, additional approval from a foreign embassy or consulate may be required; this can be in the form of a letter from the consulate.[23] The International Narcotics Control Board has information about individual countries and traveling with controlled substances (https://www.incb.org/incb/en/travellers/country-regulations.html).[24] Some medications have trade or generic names that are not registered with the International Nonproprietary Name and thus will not be used appropriately. When supplying medications to patients, you may be doing more harm than good if the patient does not have continuous access to these medications or if these medications do not exist in the country. Patients may find that a medicine may go against their religious or cultural beliefs (ie, pork-based heparin in some Muslim countries). Providers should make patient-centered decisions when prescribing medications abroad and follow in-country standard treatment recommendations.

Safety

Safety of yourself and others is a priority when traveling internationally. Thus, it is important to understand travel risks and prepare for the challenges ahead. When traveling from the United States, it is recommended to subscribe to Travel.State.Gov (https://travel.state.gov/content/travel.html) and enroll in the Smart Traveler Enrollment Program (STEP) to receive safety and security information both before and during an international trip. Review these travel advisory resources before an international departure.[25]

During international travel, it is suggested.

- Always stay with a group.
- Be aware of your surroundings and have an exit plan.
- Create a buddy system with a trusted team member.
- Be aware of curfews, and when possible, avoid traveling at night.
- Do not attract attention unnecessarily.

- Seek advice from a trusted team member/organization leader on which areas to avoid.
- Follow local news and update your family and/or friends daily.
- Having a personal locator beacon such as the *"Find My Friends"* App or other authorized personal protective devices is highly recommended.

Evacuation Planning

Many providers believe safe traveling with an NGO and may let their guard down. Remember that although the NGO may have the setting relatively under control, situations may change rapidly. Injuries, sickness, exacerbation of a preexisting condition, political instability, or an introduction of conflict may upend the best of plans. Evacuation insurance should be taken out for every trip, including aeromedical transportation. Check with your personal insurance company to see if you are covered. Additional plans may need to be purchased, and the fine print must always be closely read. Some insurance will not cover you if you are hiking, in the mountains, near water, or even just near a conflict zone. In some countries, socialized medicine may cover you, but one should not rely on this. Certain countries require payment that could be in the upward of thousands of dollars before performing an operation or CT scan.[23]

If you are in a remote area, one may need to carry a beacon, a portable device that sends a signal to a satellite allowing others to know your GPS coordinates. Consulates and embassies have registration programs, and you should register with the appropriate one. The United States has the STEP program.

Evacuation may not be specific to you. You may need to evacuate a patient. Ask if the NGO has local ground contacts for emergencies and write those numbers down. Have a plan: can a helicopter land? Will an ambulance be deployed? Is water rescue needed? One should always ensure they have a plan for themselves and their patients in case of an emergency.

WORKING WITH LIMITED RESOURCES

In many medical settings, you may work in austere environments. There are limited resources and support. These challenges are both emotional and physical, but "Do No Harm" should be a priority for all health care providers.[26] Be prepared to improvise, use supplies sparingly and rely on your history and physical examination skills (**Box 1**). Laboratory tests and diagnostic imaging may not be available. Patient communication, education, and knowledge about the country and the community are critical.

Personal Care

Providers should always recognize their limits. Working with NGOs can mean long hours. You are not in your own bed, eating food you are not accustomed to, and likely being in a different time zone. Being open and honest with your fellow team members is important. Stress and burnout are not uncommon. It can be challenging to work in an area where you see injustice and suffering. Providers often suffer from compassion fatigue and forget to take care of themselves. Providers may experience anger, isolation, frustration, and irritation, which can also be very difficult for the other team members to witness. A provider should recognize that there will always be work to be done and that they cannot fix everything. Providers need to recognize their strengths and weaknesses and ask for help. Knowing when you need a break to eat or hydrate is not a sign of weakness. Your goal is to do no harm to the population that you are helping, so you must be at your best. During deployments, find a routine, take time

---

Box 1
International American Academy of Physician Associates guidelines

HP-3700.3.0 International: AAPA International Guidelines
  HP-3700.3.1: Guidelines for PAs Working Internationally
    1. PAs should establish and maintain the appropriate physician–PA team.
    2. PAs should accurately represent their skills, training, professional credentials, identity, or service both directly and indirectly.
    3. PAs should provide only those services for which they are qualified via their education and/or experiences and in accordance with all pertinent legal and regulatory processes.
    4. PAs should respect the culture, values, beliefs, and expectations of the patients, local health care providers, and the local health care systems.
    5. PAs should be aware of the role of the traditional healer and support a patient's decision to use such care.
    6. PAs should take responsibility for being familiar with and adhering to the customs, laws, and regulations of the country where they will be providing services.
    7. When applicable, PAs should identify and train local personnel who can assume the role of providing care and continuing the education process.
    8. PA students require the same supervision abroad as they do domestically.
    9. PAs should provide the best standards of care and strive to maintain quality abroad.
    10. Sustainable programs that integrate local providers and supplies should be the goal.
    11. PAs should assign medical tasks to nonmedical volunteers only when they have the competency and supervision needed for the tasks for which they are assigned.

AAPA, American Academy of Physician Associates, guidelines as adopted by the House of Delegates, adopted 2001, reaffirmed 2006, amended 2011, reaffirmed 2016

American Academy of Physician Assistants. 2023-2024 Policy Manual - HP-6240. Published 2023. Retrieved from https://www.aapa.org/download/116915/?tmstv=1690405277.

---

for yourself, even if it is just to sit on top of a hill for 5 minutes, maintain good food, hygiene, and sleep habits. Most importantly, providers should seek help from their teammates and supervisor if they feel they are under stress or witness others under stress.[23,27,28]

Cultural Values

Culture is defined as "*customary beliefs, social forms, and material traits of a racial, religion, or social group.*"[29] Culture can include language, customs, values, and gender (if influenced by customary beliefs).[30] In the twenty-first century, there has been a growing global cultural diversity in health care and health care providers must understand how culture affects health care and the interaction to better serve patients. Health care providers must practice cultural humility.

Table 5
Cultural considerations

Ramadan: Daytime Fasting	Cannot Take certain Medications
Same-sex provider	For all examinations, not just sensitive examinations
Males as the medical authority	All medical decisions should be run through the eldest male
Dress	Appropriate coverings may be warranted
Eye contact	Considered intermuscular
Touch	Permission may be warranted

Box 2
Global Health opportunities

- PAs for Global Health become a member and get access to lists of organizations that offer PAs global opportunities as well as disaster registries www.pasforglobalhealth.com
- International Federation of Physician Assistant/Physician Associate/Clinical Officer/Clinical Associate and Comparable Student Association (IFPACS) become involved in the student organization as a mentor or student #IfPACSruledtheworld. Www.IFPACS.org
- Join the International PA Organization annual meeting at or around the time of the American Academy of Physician Assistant conference. www.internationalpas.org

---

But what is cultural humility? Cultural humility is the *"ability to maintain an interpersonal stance that is other-oriented (or open to the other) in relation to aspects of cultural identity that are most important to the [person]."*[31,32] It is an awareness of how one's culture can impact health and medical perceptions. When health care providers participate in medical humanitarian aid, they should be acquainted with and accustomed to the host country's culture. The knowledge of culture will allow culturally sensitive care.

Cultural norms such as eye contact and touch/same-sex providers are essential to recognize and understand. Before embarking on humanitarian aid, research the host

---

Box 3
Where do comparable PA descriptions exist?

Afghanistan: Physician Assistant	Germany: Physician Assistant	Mauritius: Community Health Care Officer	Sierra Leone: Community Health Officer
Angola: Clinical Officer	Ghana: Physician Assistant	Myanmar: Health Officer	South Africa: Clinical Associate
Australia: Physician Assistant	Guinea Bissau: Clinical Officer	Namibia: Clinical Officer	South Sudan: Clinical Officer
Bangladesh: Medical Assistant	Guyana: Medical Extension Officer	Nigeria: Community Health Officer	Taiwan: Physician Associate
Burkina Faso: Clinical Officer	India: Physician Assistant	Nepal: Health Assistant	Tanzania: Assistant Medical Officer
Burundi: Clinical Officer	Ireland: Physician Associate	Netherlands: Physician Assistant	Togo: Medical Assistant
Bulgaria: Physician Assistant	Israel: Physician Assistant	New Zealand: Physician Associate	Tonga: Health Officer
Canada: Physician Assistant	Kenya: Clinical Officer	Papua New Guinea: Health Extension Officer	Uganda: Clinical Officer UK: Physician Associate
Cape Verde: Health Officer	Laos: Medical Assistant	Russia: Feldsher	United States: Physician Assistant
China: Medical Officer	Liberia: Physician Assistant	Rwanda: Clinical Officer	Zambia: Clinical Officer or Medical Licentiate
Ethiopia: Health Officer or Emergency Surgical Officer	Malaysia: Assistant Medical Officer Malawi: Clinical Officer	Saudi Arabia: Physician Assistant Senegal: Health Officer	Zimbabwe: Health Officer
Gabon: Clinical Officer			

PA is used for both Physician Assistant and Physician Associate.

Source: Showstark M, Hix LR, Kereto L, John S, Uakkas S, Berkowitz O. IFPACS: Creating a Global Federation of Physician Assistant and Comparable Students. J physician Assist Educ Off J Physician Assist Educ Assoc. 2021;32(1):65-69. doi:10.1097/JPA.0000000000000346

Box 4
PA comparable reciprocity

Currently, reciprocity for PAs is a complex situation: please contact PAs for Global Health (www. pasforglobalhealth.com) for additional information/questions.

For the United States, as per the Accreditation Review Commission on Education for the Physician Assistant, Inc (ARC-PA)[34]

"The ARC-PA accredits only qualified PA programs offered by, or located within, institutions chartered by and physically located within, the United States and where students are geographically located within the United States for their education."

---

country's history, language (eg, common phrases and greetings), acceptable dress codes/customs, diet, family dynamics/communications, religious holidays, and beliefs toward Western medical practices and herbal treatments. For example, in some developing countries, it is cheaper to buy rice, so asking a patient to increase the amount of fruits and vegetables in their diet to manage diabetes may be impossible. Having a poor cultural understanding can lead to poor health outcomes and patient dissatisfaction.[33] Contact the participating organization and speak to the team about their experiences (**Table 5**) (**Boxes 2–4**).

SUMMARY

Health care providers should be adaptable, recognize their strengths and weaknesses, and ask for help when needed. It is imperative to work as a team when abroad. Communication is crucial, and providers should strive to learn from, with, and about each other and their patients. Providers must incorporate the cultural needs of a community. Research before embarking on an international humanitarian aid mission and accepting personal accountability is vital. Providers must be willing to work outside their standard routine work but should not practice outside of their scope of practice. Medical supplies and medications needed may differ in each country, and the provider must know the specific rules for their destination. Personal self-care and provider burnout should be monitored closely. There is always aid needed in the world and a role for the provider. Offering yourself and your services to a medical mission is a selfless act with many rewards. Being prepared will help the trip go smoothly and make for a great experience.

PEARL AND PITFALLS

Pearls

- maximum good for the maximum number of patients in the shortest time with the available resources is the key to triage
- using physical examination skills in remote regions that do not have diagnostics
- using medications and supplies sparingly
- learning to improvise but still providing the best care possible

Pitfalls

- not devising an evacuation plan
- not learning about the culture before entering the country
- not recognizing your personal boundaries
- creating a parallel health system (see above)

ADDITIONAL RESOURCES

1. https://wwwnc.cdc.gov/travel
2. https://travel.state.gov/content/travel.html
3. https://step.state.gov/(Smart Traveler Enrollment Program)
4. https://travel.state.gov/content/travel/en/international-travel/before-you-go/travelers-checklist.html
5. https://www.wango.org/resources.aspx?section=ngodir
6. https://www.pasforglobalhealth.com
7. http://msf.org
8. http://hopkinshumanitarianhealth.org/education/help-course/= https://handbook.spherestandards.org/en/sphere/#ch001

ACKNOWLEDGMENTS

The article would not be possible without the help and support of Physician Assistants for Global Health or PAGH or PAs.

DISCLOSURE

The views/opinions expressed are those of the authors and do not represent the views of the Yale School of Medicine or the National Commission on Certification of Physician Assistants (NCCPA). No other relevant disclosures or conflicts of interest exist. The authors are board members of Physician Assistants/Associates for Global Health (PAGH). Showstark is the Global Ambassador to the AAPA, Liaison to Euro-PAC, Communications Director for the International Association of Physician Assistant Educators, and creator of the International Federation of PAs/Clinical Officers/Clinical Associates and Comparable Student Organization.

REFERENCES

1. Haug H. The Fundamental Principles of the international red Cross and red Crescent movement - ICRC. Paul Haupt Pulishers; 1993. Available at: https://www.icrc.org/en/doc/resources/documents/publication/p2116-03.htm. Accessed August 16, 2020.
2. Wilkinson P. In: Wilkinson P, editor. Intergovernmental organizations (IGOs). 1st ed. Oxford University Press; 2007. https://doi.org/10.1093/actrade/9780192801579.003.0004.
3. Sethia B, Kumar P. Essentials of global health. 1st ed. Elsevier; 2018. Available at:.
4. Karns MP, Mingst KA, Stiles KW. International organizations: the politics and processes of global governance. 3rd. Edition. Lynne Rienner Publishers; 2015. Available at: https://www.rienner.com/uploads/55b14c992d1b2.pdf.
5. The World Bank. What We Do. Available at: https://www.worldbank.org/en/what-we-do. Accessed August 15, 2020.
6. Harman S, Wenham C. Governing Ebola: between global health and medical humanitarianism. Globalizations 2018;15(3):362–76.
7. Spiegel P, Chanis R, Scognamiglio T, et al. Innovative humanitarian health financing for refugees. Heal Policy Syst Responses to Forced Migr 2018;16(90):35–52.
8. Spiegel PB. The humanitarian system is not just broke, but broken: Recommendations for future humanitarian action. Lancet 2017;6736(17):1–8.
9. OECD. Paris Declaration and Accra Agenda for Action. Available at: https://www.oecd.org/dac/effectiveness/parisdeclarationandaccraagendaforaction.htm. Accessed July 24, 2020.

10. Norton I, von Schreeb J, Aitken P, et al. Classification and Minimum Standards for Foreign Medical Teams in Sudden Onset Disasters; 2013. Available at: http://www.who.int/hac/global_health_cluster/fmt_guidelines_september2013.pdf?ua=1. Accessed July 24, 2020.

11. UNDP. Sustainable Development Goals. Published 2023. Accessed July 24, 2020. Available at: https://www.undp.org/sustainable-development-goals.

12. UNDP. Background of the Sustainable Development Goals. Accessed July 24, 2020. Available at: https://www.undp.org/sdg-accelerator/background-goals.

13. World Health Organization. Sustainable Development Goals. United Nations Foundation. Accessed August 16, 2020. Available at: https://unfoundation.org/what-we-do/issues/sustainable-development-goals/?gclid=Cj0KCQjwsuP5BR CoARIsAPtX_wEdN6KpA_5nsmlTEeGk3qmjm00lgBwvGl_pihiGpUh6d7Hf7o4XB iMaAm3fEALw_wcB.

14. Social Determinants of Health | CDC. Available at: https://www.cdc.gov/about/sdoh/index.html. Accessed August 23, 2023.

15. Bennett NM, Brown MT, Medical A et al. Addressing Social Determinants of Health (SDOH): Beyond the Clinic WallsImprove health outcomes by addressing social determinants of health. Publ online 201821.

16. Raifman MA, Raifman JR. Disparities in the Population at Risk of Severe Illness From COVID-19 by Race/Ethnicity and Income. Am J Prev Med 2020;59(1): 137–9.

17. Artiga S, Hinton E. Beyond health care: the role of social determinants in Promoting health and health equity. Kaiser Family Foundation; 2018. Available at: https://www.kff.org/racial-equity-and-health-policy/issue-brief/beyond-health-care-the-role-of-social-determinants-in-promoting-health-and-health-equity/. Accessed August 20, 2023.

18. CDC. Pack smart. Travelers' Health; 2019. Available at: https://wwwnc.cdc.gov/travel/page/pack-smart. Accessed July 31, 2020.

19. The International Society of Travel Medicine. Available at: https://www.istm.org. Accessed August 23, 2023.

20. World Health Organization. Guidelines for Medicine Donations Revised 2010. 2011. Available at: https://www.who.int/publications-detail-redirect/978924150 1989. Accessed August 23, 2023.

21. WHO | Donations *of medicines and medical devices*, 2015, WHO. Available at: https://www.who.int/teams/health-product-and-policy-standards/medicines-selection-ip-and-affordability/donations. Accessed August 23, 2023.

22. Traveling Abroad with Medicine | Travelers' Health | CDC. Available at: https://wwwnc.cdc.gov/travel/page/travel-abroad-with-medicine. Accessed August 23, 2023.

23. Showstark M. Serving the Underserved Internationally. Physician Assist Clin 2019;4(1). https://doi.org/10.1016/j.cpha.2018.08.015.

24. Country regulations for travellers carrying medicines Containing controlled substances. International Narcotics Control Board; 2022. Available at: https://www.incb.org/incb/en/travellers/country-regulations.html. Accessed August 25, 2023.

25. U.S. Department of State. Smart Traveler Enrollment Program A SERVICE OF THE BUREAU OF CONSULAR AFFAIRS. Available at: https://step.state.gov. Accessed August 23, 2023.

26. Chen HY, Ahmad CA, Lim Abdullah K. Disaster relief work: The experiences of volunteers in Malaysia. Int J Disaster Risk Reduct 2020;43:101414.

27. Asgary R, Lawrence K. Characteristics, determinants and perspectives of experienced medical humanitarians: a qualitative approach. BMJ Open 2014;4(12). https://doi.org/10.1136/bmjopen-2014.

28. Jachens L, Houdmont J, Thomas R. Effort–reward imbalance and burnout among humanitarian aid workers. Disasters 2019;43(1):67–87.

29. Merriam-Webster Dictionary. Culture Definition and Meaning. https://www.merriam-webster.com/dictionary/culture. Accessed August 20, 2021.

30. Hughes V, Delva S, Nkimbeng M, et al. Not missing the opportunity: Strategies to promote cultural humility among future nursing faculty. J Prof Nurs 2020;36(1): 28–33.

31. Hook JN, Davis DE, Owen J, et al. Cultural humility: Measuring openness to culturally diverse clients. J Couns Psychol 2013;60(3):353–66.

32. Sykes KJ. Short-term medical service trips: A systematic review of the evidence. Am J Public Health 2014;104(7):38–48.

33. Juckett G. Cross-Cultural Medicine. Vol 72.; 2005. http://www.depts.washington. Accessed August 10, 2020.

34. Accreditation Review Commission on Education for the Physician Assistant. Accreditation Standards for Physician Assistant Education. Published 2019. https://www.arc-pa.org/accreditation/standards-of-accreditation/. Accessed August 2, 2020.

Editorial

Sacred Valley Health: Health Promotion Through Sustainability

KEY WORDS

- Community health worker • Peru • Health promotion • Sustainability
- Community partnership • Health equity

KEY POINTS

- Sacred Valley Health is a nonprofit operating a Community Health Worker program in rural Peru.
- Sustainability is key to health promotion in underserved areas.
- Community partnerships are essential to sustainability.
- Community Partnered Participatory Research methods positively contribute to health education efficacy and equity.

INTRODUCTION

Sacred Valley Health (SVH) is a community-based, public health nonprofit that partners with vibrant, indigenous communities in the Andes of Peru. Founded in 2012, the core purpose of SVH is to improve the health and well-being of these underserved, marginalized communities. SVH has developed a community health worker (CHW) program that empowers local women's education, resources, professional development, and economic opportunities. This community partner approach, working *with* remote communities to increase health care and knowledge, has a secondary purpose: it provides vocational training to women and elevates them as leaders within their communities. Many global medical outreach programs are limited, in both resources and time, to sustain medical outreach. SVH in Peru has solved this issue by training local women with a culturally relevant CHW program. The curriculum has been developed and refined by the local CHW experts allowing for collaboration with international partners. Having the local experts teach the international medical volunteers provides a bidirectional global health learning opportunity.

GEOGRAPHIC, CULTURAL, AND SOCIOECONOMIC CONTEXT

In the Sacred Valley of Peru, indigenous Quechua communities are located high in the Andes Mountains: 9500 to 13,500 feet above sea level. Communities are dependent on local government health clinics for their health care needs. These clinics, which provide only basic care and limited resources for current health information, may be 30 minutes

Physician Assist Clin 9 (2024) 243–251
https://doi.org/10.1016/j.cpha.2023.11.006
2405-7991/24/© 2023 Elsevier Inc. All rights reserved.

to 3 hours away by car. Transportation is inconsistent, unreliable, and, in some cases, nonexistent. Weather, roadblocks, and/or poor road conditions can make this journey even more difficult. Many people travel most of this distance on foot over rugged mountain terrain.

These communities are just as far from fresh food markets, presenting access barriers to nutritional needs for all ages. In these high-altitude communities, residents practice subsistence farming to augment seasonal income from tourism-related work. This remoteness has led to high rates of poverty and preventable illnesses: malnutrition, respiratory disease, or pregnancy and maternal health issues. Culturally sensitive health care, especially for women, is even more scarce. In this society, women are traditionally the family caretakers. When women experience illness, they are unable to care for their families, and when family members are sick, women have few resources to care for them.

To further compound these barriers, indigenous women are disproportionately affected by poverty and have fewer opportunities for vocational education than men. Access to schools is very limited due to their remoteness. Men are generally given preference when opportunities for high school and post–high school education do arise, whereas women are expected to leave school early to assist with household duties or start families of their own. Gender discrimination means women often end up in insecure, low-wage jobs, or doing unpaid, intensive home labor.

In Peru's Sacred Valley, women from Quechua-speaking communities are usually financially dependent on their husbands. The few opportunities that do exist for women are difficult to access due to geographic and language barriers. Traditionally, Quechua-speaking communities have an oral culture where teaching and learning happen through word, story, song, and action, rather than through reading and writing. As a result, literacy levels in Spanish, the dominant language in Peru, among indigenous women remain low. Most educational institutions do not teach the local language and culture, creating barriers to education and the understanding of health information.

HISTORY OF SCARED VALLEY HEALTH

In January 2010, Keri Baker, RN, a long-term medical volunteer, was in Ollantaytambo to develop a health program to meet the needs of local communities. In 2011, while volunteering at a local mountain community, Keri was approached by a community member regarding a young woman too sick to leave her home. The woman had received treatment for an infection 1 month earlier at a local clinic. However, she stopped her antibiotics due to side effects. The infection progressed, and she was now unable to walk without pain. However, she was unable to afford transportation for a second clinic visit. After taking the patient to the clinic for treatment, Keri realized this was not an unusual case. Keri recognized the root cause of the issue and the need for affordable and effective local health care. This was the inspiration to create a mobile health clinic.

Keri and Dr Mark Willcox, both volunteers in the Ollantaytambo district, began a monthly mobile clinic in 2011. The clinic was so popular that the local government adapted the concept and started its own mobile clinic visiting communities in 2012. Mark and Keri, along with Sarah FitzGerald and Emily Groves, shifted their focus to a more integrated, sustainable approach—a CHW program, and in 2012, SVH was founded. SVH would complement rather than compete with the local government's efforts. In consultation with organizations running similar, successful programs in other parts of Peru, SVH started a CHW program specific for this region of Peru. By educating, empowering, and employing local women while collaborating with communities, SVH is able to integrate the biomedical model for health education with indigenous knowledge in a culturally competent way.

TRANSITION TO SUSTAINABILITY

SVH launched their CHW program, locally known as *promotoras de salud*, to improve health. A side benefit would be empowering the local population to improve health in these underserved, indigenous communities. It was important that this program include not only education but also collaboration and cultural competency. The CHWs, 97% of whom are women, are elected by their communities and act as health educators and promoters; they help with early detection and health care referrals. They serve as health advocates and leaders for sustainable community-wide changes via home visits and/or community-wide presentations. CHWs also initiate health-focused projects for their home communities (**Fig. 1**).

PROGRAMMING

The CHW training consists of three distinct and complementary programs covering health, education, access, empowerment, and economic agency. The basis and foundation CHW Program is the *Promotora* Program, a 2-year training focused on fundamental learning techniques, leadership, health education, and individual behavior change. CHWs receive monthly training on specific health topics (hygiene, water purification, nutrition, reproductive health, communicable and noncommunicable disease, and first aid). Between the monthly trainings, CHWs are visited in their home communities by *docentes*. *Docentes* are advanced CHWs paid by SVH as trainers and supervisors. The *docentes* help professionally support the new CHWs as they perform community work (**Fig. 2**).

CHWs receive a bag of healthy food incentives at each training and free meals on training days and are compensated for community work based on the number of house visits and community presentations completed.

The second step in SVH's CHW program is the *Graduate Promotora* Program. The Graduate Program is continuing education and professional development for CHWs who are actively working in their communities. At this level, CHWs receive more

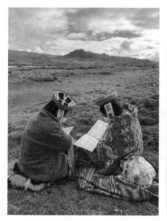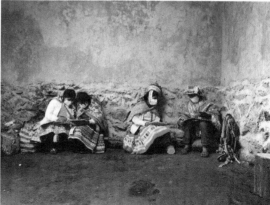

Fig. 1. CHWs study their curriculum at a training session. (*Photo credit: Kathryn Arone and Nicole Weber.*)

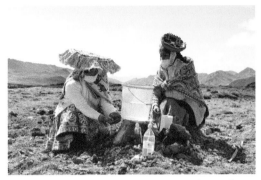

Fig. 2. Docente Matiasa teaches handwashing to CHWs in the Andean community of Challwaccocha. (*Photo credit: Kathryn Arnone.*)

advanced training to consider the community as the patient. CHWs examine how society, community infrastructure, and access to resources impact the health of individuals and communities at large. The CHWs learn community asset mapping and community mobilization. Over the course of the program, the CHWs plan and implement a community health project. The *Graduate Promotora* students still receive support and guidance from *docentes* and local staff as well as funding for project implementation. Graduate CHWs also have the opportunity to participate in certification programs that focus on specific topics like women's health, nutrition, and advanced first aid.

The highest level of CHW is the *Docente. Docente* means teacher in Spanish, and in the "train-the-trainer" program, CHWs can apply for and train to become paid part-time *docente* employees. Once hired, these women receive monthly workshops on leadership, teaching, program development, and advanced levels of health information. They prepare and facilitate CHW trainings, provide CHWs with support and supervision in their communities, and assist with evaluation activities and office work. All *docentes* participate in monthly professional development activities and assist with office tasks. All *docentes* receive a monthly salary and benefits—a first for most women participating in this program. The three-level training program works to provide women with pay, professional development, and leadership opportunities, showing the women in the community that they can be leaders.

COMMUNITY PARTNERSHIPS

SVH has partnered with local communities to develop, implement, and evaluate the CHW program. In order to ensure sustainability of local CHWs, SVH used the *docentes*, CHWs, local staff, and community leaders to assist in developing educational programs that best fit local culture, language, available resources, and traditional health practices. This is referred to as the Community Partnered Participatory Research (CPPR) method. Using CPPR, SVH has developed a subspecialty CHW subprogram in advanced nutrition and women's health. The CMWs have even developed a personal development program for local adolescent girls.

CURRICULUM DEVELOPMENT

SVH's curriculum is customized for and cocreated by indigenous, Quechua-speaking health workers. The curriculum requires approval from local, Quechua-speaking staff at every step, ensuring all levels of CHWs are well versed in program development. By providing high-quality, culturally relevant education and resources based on the local learning methodology, the hope is to have this program sustain itself in the long run. SVH uses a local graphic designer to design images for the curriculum guide to ensure each topic is effective and accessible. Teaching activities use storytelling (an important aspect of the local culture) and discussion to prompt problem solving. Previously, lessons were focused on individual behavior change but were not effective; by moving to community-based interventions (problem-solving for each person and community), outreach education is more effective (**Figs. 3 and 4**).

This sustainable approach to curriculum development has been an invaluable initiative for the SVH local Peruvian staff, who comprises the majority of the curriculum development team. The staff started as CHWs and worked their way up to their permanent, full-time management positions. The staff has focused primarily on teaching, supervising, and providing final consultation on curriculum. The curriculum was developed from the ground up (rather than top down), and this provides consistency and sustainability in SVH programs. Foreign SVH staff and volunteers may come and go, so it is important the local staff has the skills necessary to plan, implement, and evaluate programs. Their unique knowledge and skills ensure that this fits local needs and culture. This approach to curriculum development is more effective than a top-down method. Average test scores for first-year CHWs in 2016 were 56% for the curriculum developed by outsiders. After the local curriculum revision, this improved to 96% for first-year CHWs.

MONITORING AND EVALUATION

SVH aims to improve health through health education and promotion for both the individual and the community. As is important for any nonprofit enterprise, SVH tracks

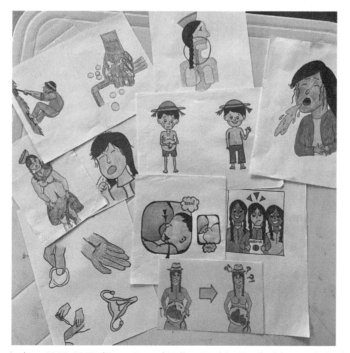

Fig. 3. Curriculum 2014–2017. (*From* Sacred Valley Health. Used with permission)

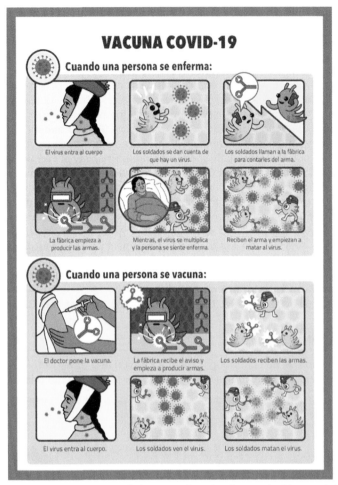

Fig. 4. Curriculum 2022. (*Courtesy of* Alexis Loyola Delgado. Used with permission)

progress of the health education and promotion program activities. They wish to show that a CHW changes knowledge, attitudes, beliefs, and practices that then improve health outcomes. SVH's CHW program attempts to shift power from outsiders to the local population. Methods are person- and culture-centric rather than number-centric (**Fig. 5**).

Because it is important for the local leaders to see change in their community, they provide the system, process, and structure for the ideas, desires, goals, and skills brought to the table. The goal is to transition from community "*buy-in*" to community ownership. SVH uses pretests and posttests to assess knowledge transfer to CHWs during trainings, comprehensive evaluations to assess knowledge and skill retention, field observation, work documentation, community surveys, and focus groups to measure the success of its programming and guide necessary changes for more effective service delivery.

OUTCOMES

- The number of active SVH CHWs has grown from 11 in 2012 to 54 in 2023 (*a 79% increase*).

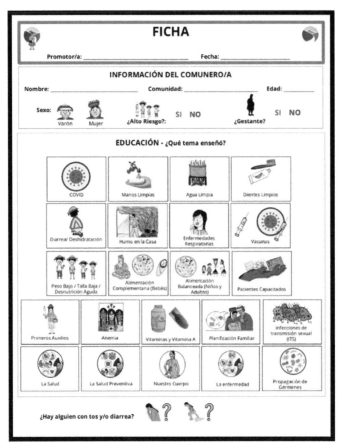

Fig. 5. Work documentation. (*From* Sacred Valley Health. Used with permission.)

- The number of local staff has grown from 2 in 2012 to 9 in 2023 (*a 78% increase*).
- The number of house visits made by CHWs has increased from 160 in 2012 to 4370 in 2023 (*a 96% increase*).
- Of community members who have received a visit from a CHW, 82% are able to recall at least one fact they learned from an SVH CHW (*according to community health profile data collected by SVH in May 2022*).
- During focus group evaluations with CHWs conducted in June 2022, CHWs identified their participation at health education trainings and their ability to apply what they've learned as the two most beneficial aspects of being a CHW.
- During focus group evaluations with CHWs employed as *docentes* in SVH's train-the-trainer program conducted in June 2022, 100% of *docentes* (all women) reported that they feel more empowered because of their vocational training with SVH. They identified the following benefits as an employee at SVH:
  ○ Receiving a salary, allowing them to provide for their families
  ○ Increased knowledge
  ○ Assuming more leadership within their community
  ○ Improved skills and confidence in public speaking

SUSTAINABILITY DURING COVID-19

The COVID-19 pandemic exacerbated preexisting barriers to health, and it had a devastating impact on all of Peru. The communities, remote to begin with, were even more isolated because of national quarantine mandates. Inconsistent communication about the virus, constantly changing government regulations, and limited education about prevention negatively impacted health outcomes. Compounding the health crisis, Peru suffered one of the worst economic contractions in South America. According to the World Bank, the pandemic forced an additional 2 million Peruvians into poverty. The main source of income in the Cusco region is tourism, which was nonexistent for 2 years. This meant for many families that their household income disappeared entirely while disrupted supply chains caused the prices of necessities to grow exponentially.

Although the pandemic created barriers and increased isolation for these communities, it also increased interest among community members to learn about health, illness, and prevention methods from their CHWs. This, in turn, meant people were inclined to adopt new health behaviors. It demonstrated the importance and effectiveness of prevention behaviors and community systems that support the whole population. In addition, it highlighted the resources present in these Andean communities, where traditional agriculture practices, indigenous knowledge of plant medicine, and a much more sustainable way of life contributed to these communities' ability to endure months of isolation, lockdowns, and disrupted supply chains.

SVH adapted its training curriculum by increasing information regarding immunity and vaccinations and adding a chapter on COVID-19. Training was also adapted; instead of coming to SVH headquarters for monthly trainings, a small team of program staff and *docentes* traveled to communities to safely teach smaller groups in outdoor settings.

SUSTAINABILITY THROUGH INTERNATIONAL PARTNERSHIP

An overarching goal is to develop a permanent funding arm to generate enough money for SVH's operations. Prior to COVID-19, SVH was moving from a service model (students groups come to Peru to carry out service projects) to a system where students, health professionals, and other visitors come to learn about health and practices in the local culture, where they can learn from the locals rather than teaching the locals how things are done outside of the local community. This program provides current and future health professionals with an ethical global health learning experience that emphasizes local voices as teachers in a practical setting.

The advantages of the local teaching the outsider include the following:

1. *Participatory approaches*: Understanding the importance of local input at all stages of program development and implementation.
2. *Cultural exchange*: Promoting ethical cultural exchange between visiting groups, CHWs, and partner communities.
3. Preserving local wisdom, culture, and practices by creating spaces for that knowledge to be shared and celebrated.
4. Empowering local women and communities by highlighting them as experts and teachers in local community health perspectives.
5. *Economic empowerment*: Providing opportunities for communities and CHWs to earn income by facilitating and hosting groups of students and tourists.
6. Contributing to the financial sustainability of SVH and increasing organizational capacity by generating unrestricted income for CHW programs.

CLINICAL IMPLICATIONS

Wilderness medicine is practiced in austere areas; this is never truer than the small villages of the Andes. Although the work carried out by SVH does not take place in a clinical setting, the clinical implications are vast. Sustainable models for health promotion broadens the lens through which practitioners can view health:

- It is important to understanding the cultural, social, and economic context that contribute to a presenting health problem. Barriers to health are just as important as medication.
- Sometimes, a bottom-up teaching method is more effective.
- It is important to involve the full health care team, and most importantly, patients themselves as fellow *collaborators* in the creation of their health plan.
- Language impacts the way one perceives, treats, and interacts with people, communities, and cultures.
- Health promotion in an international setting should be provided in an ethical, sustainable, collaborative way.

To learn more about Sacred Valley Health, please visit www.sacredvalleyhealth.org/.

DISCLOSURE

The authors have nothing to disclose.

Jenny Jordan, RN, BSN
Sacred Valley Health
Pilochuasi s/n
Ollantaytambo, Cusco, Peru

Audra Baca, MPH, CHES

Keri Baker, MS, MSN, ENP, FNP-C

E-mail addresses:
JJordan@sacredvalleyhealth.org (J. Jordan)
Audrabaca@outlook.com (A. Baca)
Kbaker@sacredvalleyhealth.org (K. Baker)

Introduction to the Wilderness

Seth C. Hawkins, MD, W/NR-EMT[a,b,c,*]

KEYWORDS

- Wilderness medicine • Wilderness EMS • Search and rescue • Wilderness • EMS

KEY POINTS

- Wilderness is more defined by geography and less defined by access to outside assistance.
- Wilderness medicine may be practiced by any clinician who assists in natural disasters; from hurricanes to fires to volcanos to mud slides to tsunamis, etc.
- Wilderness medicine has moved from a frequently volunteer hobby to an evidence- based professional specialty and may be the most inclusive of all practices of medicine.

INTRODUCTION

Medical care outside the traditional environment, including care outside of clinics and other facilities, is one of the most fertile and rewarding contexts where practitioners can apply their medical knowledge and skills. When this work is outside traditional or front country Emergency Medical Services (EMS), it is often categorized as expedition medicine, wilderness medicine, or wilderness EMS. Opportunities abound to work in these spaces.

DEFINITIONS

Wilderness medicine in the past was defined in terms of time to definitive care (usually and somewhat arbitrarily 1–2 hours) but this approach proved operationally problematic. When the clock started and stopped for this definition was not clear, how a clinician or other operator could prospectively know how long an operation would take was not clear and the definition of *definitive care* was not clear. Every key element of such a definition was problematic.

In other formulations, *wilderness medicine* is defined as care in resource-deficient environments. However, this definition fails to capture those cases in which wilderness

[a] Department of Emergency Medicine, Wake Forest University, Medical Center Boulevard, Winston-Salem, NC 27157-1089, USA; [b] Department of Anthropology, Wake Forest, Winston-Salem, NC, USA; [c] NC Department of Natural and Cultural Resources, (State Parks)
* Corresponding author.
E-mail address: schawkin@wakehealth.edu

Physician Assist Clin 9 (2024) 253–260
https://doi.org/10.1016/j.cpha.2023.11.004
2405-7991/24/© 2023 Elsevier Inc. All rights reserved.

physicianassistant.theclinics.com

medical operations actually have more, or at least different, resources than other types of medical care. Wilderness medical operations can include helicopters that are not available even for care of patients in emergency departments, both in terms of time of availability (ex: storms) and type of platform (ex: military or hoist-equipped helicopters). Wilderness medical operations can include specialized tools such as Gamow bags and self contained under water breathing apparatus (SCUBA) gear which, rather than being resource deficient, in fact represent a cutting edge of expensive and sophisticated technology. Many examples of such medical care and equipment are included in this issue of *PA Clinics*. While wilderness medicine historically has a large emphasis on improvisation, and this remains important, it is not exclusively the realm of improvisation. In wilderness EMS, defined as the systematic and preplanned delivery of wilderness medicine, there are often quite high levels of resources and technology, especially in wilderness rescue or search and rescue (SAR). Outside considerations of just technology, wilderness medicine and SAR have also traditionally relied on high levels of volunteerism. In this model, volunteers for local mountain rescue teams, rescue squads, fire departments, swift water rescue teams, and other organized rescue services will volunteer their time to deliver the needed care.

Another example of a prior definition of wilderness medicine now considered to be problematic is care delivered in certain fixed locations (this river, that mountain-top, a certain canyon) or for certain conditions (lightning strikes, hypothermia, etc). The problem with fixed location-driven definitions is it ignores what the Wilderness EMS Medical Director Course has defined as the Gusteau Principle, playing off the famous Disney movie *Ratotouille* and its contention that *"anyone can cook"*; here, the contention is that *"anywhere can be a location requiring wilderness care."*[1] A common example of this is weather emergency. Hurricane Sandy in New England converted communities that would never have been considered *wilderness* into spaces requiring wilderness care. Hurricane Katrina famously turned the floors of Charity Hospital, one of the largest hospitals in one of the largest cities in the country, into a space where wilderness medicine was required.[2] The challenge with applying the term "wilderness medicine" exclusively to certain environmental conditions is that delivery of care can occur in urban areas as well as remote locations. Examples include the prevalence of lightning on golf courses or hypothermia and hyperthermia in urban centers during extreme weather conditions.

In more modern terminology, most major textbooks have adapted these definitions or a close approximation.[1,3–6]

- Wilderness (medical definition): those areas where fixed or transient geographic challenges reduce availability of, or alter requirements for, medical or patient movement resources
- Wilderness medicine: medical care delivered in those areas where fixed or transient geographic challenges reduce availability of, or alter requirements for, medical or patient movement resources
- Wilderness EMS: the systematic and preplanned delivery of wilderness medicine by trained clinicians[a]

One critical feature of these definitions is that they are fundamentally geographic (using the expanded meaning of geography beyond simply location-based), emphasizing that wilderness medicine and wilderness EMS are fundamentally geographically-

---

[a] In this article, clinician refers to all health care categories, including but not limited to EMTs, EMRs (Emergency Medical Responders), paramedics PAs, APRNs, and physicians, etc. Practitioner refers to those who have capacity independent of fixed delegated practice protocols and who have prescription writing capacity: PAs, APRNs, and physicians.[19]

determined medical specialties. This differs from a simple location-based definition by introducing the concept of *fixed or transient* geographic features, acknowledging that the same location can be wilderness or not, depending on circumstance. An example is a river in or out of flood stage or a neighborhood school or city park with or without a hurricane. The critical health care element of this definition is the presence of a patient and the delivery of medical care. The impact of the fixed or transient geographic features is on the type of equipment available and the ability to transport that patient. Transport considerations are a minor part, if any, of most medical specialties, but are central to the definition of both EMS and wilderness medicine/EMS.

HISTORY AND PHILOSOPHY

Wilderness work can occur anywhere: from cold, dark, remote to blazingly hot, bright, and urban. It can be quite physically challenging requiring ropes, hiking and/or skis, or it can be near a metro system. Sometimes, it is work in areas that are considered paradises or a recreationalist's dream. This leads to the perception that wilderness medicine is a hobby or a chance to pretend to be working while actually enjoying the landscape.

In reality, even in attractive spaces, wilderness medicine can be brutally difficult. As with any type of medical care, there can be elements which are exceptionally rewarding and other elements which require significant physical and emotional skills along with the maturity not to sustain physical or emotional stress injuries. Technologies of psychological first aid have recently been elucidated as an evidence-based way to reduce, identify, and treat psychological stress injuries. These use a first aid format and are available to and applicable by anyone.[7–9]

In the twentieth century, the recreationalist or hobbyist concept was sometimes used in marketing to promote the field of wilderness medicine. The Wilderness Medical Society (WMS), throughout much of the twentieth century, carried the tagline *"Combining Your Profession With Your Passion."*[6] However, hobbyism carried the risk of compromising the authority of health care professionals who worked in wilderness spaces versus those, often not health care professionals, who considered it a job: rangers, guides, rescue personnel, etc. Another danger of promoting hobbyism or the recreationalist elements of working as a health care professional in a wilderness environment was the idea that actual, legitimate, paying careers were not available in this space. Most health care professionals in the twentieth century interested in wilderness medicine were advised this could be pursued as a hobby but was not appropriate as a primary career.

It is true that the majority of wilderness medical care delivered by health care professionals is either within a pre-existing EMS format or not as a primary career. The Golden Age of Wilderness Medicine, starting in the late 1960s and early 1970s is when wilderness medicine first began to appear as a discrete medical specialty.[1] In the twenty firstst century, there are now numerous ways that wilderness medicine is a legitimate academic and practice track with industry-wide applications and recognitions. The WMS was founded in the 1980s as a professional medical society dedicated to medical care delivered in wilderness spaces. Subsequently, it built the Academy of Wilderness Medicine, which offers fellowship recognition in its specialty: Fellow of the Academy of Wilderness Medicine (FAWM). They also maintain a Master Fellowship (MFAWM) for individuals pursuing more advanced and individualized training. In a hallmark of wilderness medical culture and practice, this honorific is available to any clinician, not just physicians. This represents the recognition by the WMS that wilderness medicine is delivered by multiple health professionals. This contention is carried further by the horizontal hierarchy principle in wilderness medicine as proposed in the textbook *Wilderness EMS*. This philosophy argues that the vertical hierarchy found in medicine within 4 walls is non-functional and potentially even harmful when applied to wilderness spaces. In the horizontal hierarchy model, the person with the most appropriate training for a specific operation is the one to lead the team, not (in contradiction to most vertical hierarchical models) the person with the most hours of training or the higher number of credentials.[1] The horizontal hierarchy model aligns nicely with team-based care models promoted by PA and advanced practice registered nurse (APRN) societies and training. Often wilderness EMS and wilderness medicine is by necessity a team-based medical practice drawing together numerous operators and practitioners with broad and disparate training to accomplish a mission. Indeed, in a historical view of wilderness medicine, we now exist in the Evidence-Based and Collaboration Age of its practice, emphasizing the prevalence and need for team-based approaches including all types of field operators and researchers to drive the evidence for those operators.[1]

TRAINING AND EDUCATION

Promoting the new professionalism regarding wilderness medicine in the twenty first century includes numerous training pathways that exist within academia. These would not have been available from the 1960s to the 1980s. Wilderness medicine is 1 of the only 2 medical specialties (space medicine might be another) which grew up outside traditional medical academia. Currently, numerous universities have wilderness medicine student interest groups and even designated *Fellowships.* The fellowships are usually year-long experiences with a specialization in wilderness medicine. Two medical centers, University of New Mexico and Wake Forest University, have developed merged programs between wilderness medicine and EMS fellowships. These offer a 2-year track that results in a legitimate Wilderness EMS fellowship. University fellowship tracks are available to PAs and NPs, including programs at Virginia Tech-Carilion and the Medical College of Georgia-Augusta University. Some universities have certificate tracks in wilderness medicine, both for undergraduate (medical/PA/NP students) and graduate (residency) medical trainees.[10] A significant amount of wilderness medical training still occurs in professional schools that are dedicated to delivering this care outside the WMS academy. These include Wilderness Medical Outfitters (https://wildernessmedicine.com/), Stonehearth Outdoor Learning Opportunities (https://soloschools.com/), National Outdoor Leadership School (https://www.nols.edu/en/), Wilderness Medical Associates-International (https://www.wildmed.com/), and Aerie Backcountry Medicine (https://www.aeriemedicine.com/).[1] While many of these schools were quite competitive in the twentieth century, in the twenty firstst century they have become more collaborative. In the early 2010s, many of the largest schools formed the Wilderness Medical Education Collaborative, a joint venture to promote quality in wilderness medical education. This, along with the 2022 establishment of the Wilderness Paramedic credential examination by the International Board of Specialty Certifications, has created more standardization and quality metrics in an industry that historically was felt to be lacking widely agreed-upon standards. The wilderness medicine space continues to be minimally regulated even as various organizations are beginning to develop standards that are widely accepted.

As educational and credentialing opportunities expand, so do opportunities for practice. Such practice opportunities are as varied as the environments in which wilderness medicine can be practiced.

Ski patrols and mountaineering teams provide care in snow and ice environments. The National Ski Patrol (NSP) represents one of the premier ski-based organizations. It is one of the oldest wilderness EMS organizations in the country, operating off a Congressional charter since the earliest days of wilderness EMS in the twentiethth century. The Mountain Rescue Association (MRA) (https://mra.org/) represents one of the premier mountain rescue-based organizations with a half-century of history organizing medical care and operations in mountainous terrain. It has the unique claim of glaciated mountain rescues and ice rescues. Teams can be credentialed by either of these organizations in their specific operational environments. In addition, the NSP offers an Outdoor Emergency Care credential. This credential covers all 4 seasons, recognizing the expansion of NSP into non-skiing, non-winter activities in ski areas that allow year-round operations and recreational programs. These programs include mountain biking and alpine slides.

Swiftwater rescue teams provide care in rapidly moving (swift water) environments while surf lifeguard programs are in place for coastal and surf environments. A Wilderness Lifeguard training and credential has been developed by Landmark Learning (https://www.landmarklearning.org/) and Starfish Aquatics Institute (https://www.starfishaquatics.org/) that translates lifeguard skills from a pool into unregulated wilderness environments. These can include lakes, ponds, drop pools, and slow-moving water.[11] Divers Alert Network offers resources for medical emergencies experienced by divers including a 24/7 call line to help navigate dive emergencies (919–684–9111).[12] Aquatic emergencies and their wilderness medical management represent one of the most fertile growth areas for wilderness practitioners to engage from both a caregiver and public health perspective. Drowning continually represents one of the most common causes of death (especially in pediatrics) not just in outdoor environments but in all environments across the globe.[13]

Specialized teams are often needed to deliver climbing care in both mountainous and non-mountainous environments. The Mountain Rescue Association is one of the largest supporting agencies for this type of work. Climbing rescue is particularly driven by local configurations. For example, only one fully-credentialed MRA team exists in the American Southeast (the Appalachian Mountain Rescue Team) and they were only fully credentialed in 2018. Climbing rescue involves such specialized skills that health care professionals often start as climbers and then explore resources in their climbing areas and communities for rescue activities. Climbing-oriented medical care in much of the United States is often delivered by local rescue squads and fire departments. These groups can be likely sources for volunteer work for practitioners looking for engagement in climbing medicine.

Some teams primarily provide search services, with or without medical care delivered upon their arrival, and these are usually configured as search and rescue (SAR) teams. SAR teams may also have specialized training in the terrain they cover: caves vs mountains vs canyons vs rivers vs waterfalls. Caves offer particular challenges to medical rescue. Cave rescues often draw people from multiple states and a variety of teams due to their complexity. The National Cave Rescue Commission (https://caves.org/ncrc/) is an example of an organization promoting quality medical care in cave environments.

The definition of wilderness medicine and wilderness EMS can include remote care in unexpected environments: oil rigs, scientific expeditions, or rural communities. Although these are defined as wilderness mediicine, they are usually paid opportunities rather than volunteer or part time.

MEDICAL OVERSIGHT AND MEDICAL DIRECTORS

One of the most common ways that practitioners (differentiated from other clinicians[a] and operators) insert into wilderness medical teams is as medical directors or otherwise involved in the medical oversight of a team. This can be one of the most important roles for practitioners to serve in a SAR or wilderness EMS team for numerous reasons. Practitioners often have the most extensive medicine-specific training and their credentials require the most attention to evidence and primary review of the literature. This differs from other delegated practice models involving clinicians. Emergency medical technicians (EMTs) have significantly fewer hours of medical training (albeit they may have more operational or technical training) and their continuing education model does not specifically require them to keep abreast of medical literature on their own. The role of practitioners in ensuring evidence-based practices cannot be overemphasized. Numerous examples are present in the rescue community showing decades-long perpetuation of rescue practices that presuppose a medical benefit with zero evidence or often even a sensible pathophysiological model. Examples include suspension syndrome, dry drowning concerns, and long spine board application.[14–16] In an EMS model, typically emergency medical responders, EMTs, and paramedics operate in collaboration with a practitioner, whose medical license and role activates, informs and oversees their practice. This ensures quality management, quality improvements, and evidence-based medicine.

Many states do not permit PAs or APRNs to provide direct medical oversight or to serve as medical directors of delegated practice EMS clinicians. The wilderness community endorses the team-based practice model including PAs and APRNs, and would suggest that wilderness medicine and wilderness EMS operations are a prime example of places where this model is quite successful. PAs, by nature of their background and training, often have technical and operational skills that physicians may lack. Even if PAs are not permitted to serve as medical directors in a given operational environment, they can often be assistant or associate medical directors. This allows them to use their quite formidable combination of talents to the operations of the team, including from the perspective of their medical training and skills.

The simple presence of a practitioner level credential, be it MD (Doctor of Medicine), DO (Doctor of Osteopathy), PA, or APRN, should not exclude such personnel from being effective operators. There is a tendency to think such practitioners are best utilized in command or off-line roles with significant distance in both time and space from actual field response and patient care. This is short-sighted. Often a PA, physician, or APRN with exceptional medical AND operational skills might be the most important person to put at a patient's side delivering direct medical care.

We would also caution against the concept, perhaps historically valid but increasingly challenged in the modern era, that medical oversight should be delivered off-line, via protocols, rather than in person or via radio or mobile/satellite phone. Many features historically tended to push practitioners into off-line roles, including well-meaning efforts to protect the time of such health care professionals. However, as wilderness medicine and wilderness EMS expands as a legitimate specialty and less of a hobby or a part-time role, correspondingly the culture is expanding to encourage practitioner-level response in the field and to the patient. In-person response also brings the additional medical training of practitioners to bear in the field. Sidelining the most experienced and medically trained practitioner, if they have operational and environmental skills, is short-sighted.

Field response also reinforces for medical directors the challenges faced by operators. A simple leg fracture or head injury that might be easily managed in the front country can be exceptionally complicated in the wilderness. Wind, rain, cold or the noise of a waterfall, can critically compromise both operator efficacy and patient condition. Medical directors need to experience the field to fully appreciate the power that geography and environment has on medical care and problem solving.[1]

From a regulatory standpoint, practitioner field response can expand the scope of practice of an operation. In many states, dislocation reduction is beyond the scope of a paramedic and field amputation is often the purview only of practitioners. Yet either of these interventions might be critically needed in a wilderness EMS operation.

Finally, whether in the field in on-line activities or out of it in off-line oversight, practitioners, such as PAs, physicians, or APRNs, can critically advance the concept of medically-directed rescue. Notably, the original publication citing medically-directed rescue was a collaborative effort involving PAs.[17] Medically-directed rescue argues that all rescues should put medical considerations at the forefront, including technical rescue activities. It acknowledges that a human being, not a mannequin, is on the sharp end of the rope, in the litter, or being loaded into a helicopter and medical impacts of decisions around their rescue should always be considered. In the sense that wilderness EMS is fundamentally a public health consideration (addressing the population-based care of individuals in wilderness environments), medically-directed rescue is analogous to the public health principle of Health in All Policies (HiAP).[18] HiAP argues that every public policy has health-related consequences that must be considered in design and implementation. Often a physician, PA, APRN, or other clinician may be the only representative in a highly technical operation equipped to serve as a patient advocate or the only one uniquely tasked with that role. Always advocating for patients and considering the impacts on them in any operational decision can be a critical role for either a medical director or for a medically-credentialed responder.

CLINICS CARE POINTS

- Wilderness medicine and wilderness EMS are rapidly growing fields with increasing professionalism and career opportunities, and can be considered a profession and not just a hobby

- The modern definition of wilderness medicine is fundamentally geographic, rather than temporal, location-based, or condition-based and involves challenges to patient care and movement based on fixed or transient geographic considerations

- Numerous credentials, teams, and organizing bodies exist for almost any imaginable wilderness medical environment

- Key opportunities for practitioners to insert into rescue operations include establishment of a medically-directed rescue model, inclusion of evidence-based medicine into rescue operations, and roles as either collaborative medical directors (depending on regulations) or field operators

DISCLOSURE

The author has nothing to disclose. Mention of specific training programs does not indicate support.

REFERENCES

1. Hawkins SC, editor. Wilderness EMS. Philadelphia, PA: Wolters Kluwer; 2018.

2. Berggren R. Hurricane Katrina. Unexpected Necessities — Inside Charity Hospital. N Engl J Med 2005 Oct 13;353(15):1550–3.
3. Auerbach PS, Cushing TA, Harris NS. Auerbach's wilderness medicine. 7th edition. Philadelphia, PA: Elsevier; 2017.
4. Cone DC, Brice JH, Delbridge TR, et al, for National Association of EMS Physicians. Medical Oversight of EMS. In: Emergency medical services: Clinical practice and systems oversight:, 2, 3rd ed. West Sussex, UK: Wiley; 2021.
5. National Association of EMTs. Prehospital trauma life support (PHTLS). 10th ed. Burlington, MA: Jones & Bartlett Learning; 2023.
6. Wilderness Medical Society, https://wms.org, Accessed 26 September, 2023.
7. Loewenberg H, Hawkins S. Words Matter: What If Words Could Prevent Post-Traumatic Stress Disorder? Emerg Med News 2020;42(8):24–5.
8. Loewenberg H, Hawkins S, Brisson M. Words matter: a psychological first aid toolkit for PTSD. Emerg Med News 2020;42(9):31–2.
9. McGladrey L. Psychological first aid. In: Wilderness EMS. Hawkins SC. Philadelphia, PA: Wolters Kluwer; 2018.
10. Schrading WA, Battaglioli N, Drew J, et al. Core Content for Wilderness Medicine Training: Development of a Wilderness Medicine Track in an Emergency Medicine Residency. Wilderness Environ Med 2018;29(1):78–84.
11. Padgett S. Wilderness Lifeguarding, Savannah, GA: Starfish Aquatics Institute, https://www.starfishaquatics.org/wilderness-lifeguard.html, Accessed 23 September, 2023.
12. Divers Alert Network (DAN) emergency assistance, https://dan.org/health-medicine/medical-services/emergency-assistance/, Accessed 23 September, 2023.
13. Centers for Disease Control and Prevention (CDC), Drowning Facts, https://www.cdc.gov/drowning/facts/, Accessed 23 September,2023.
14. Hawkins SC, Simon RB, Bryan R, et al. Suspension syndrome: Hanging by a thread (and a rope). Emerg Med News 2017;39(7):29–30.
15. Hawkins SC, Simon RB, Beissinger JP, et al. Vertical aid: essential wilderness medicine for climbers, trekkers, and mountaineers. New York, NY: The Countryman Press; 2017.
16. Szpilman D, Sempsrott J, Webber J, et al. 'Dry drowning' and other myths. Cleve Clin J Med 2018;85(7):529–35.
17. Brown JB, Rosengart MR, Forsythe RM, et al. Not all prehospital time is equal: Influence of scene time on mortality. J Trauma Acute Care Surg 2016;81(1):93–100.
18. Centers for Disease Control and Prevention, Health in All Policies, updated 9Jun2016, https://www.cdc.gov/policy/hiap/index.html, Accessed 23 September, 2023.
19. Hawkins SC. Wilderness medicine magazine style guidelines: 2023 edition. Austin, TX: Wilderness Medical Society. Wilderness Medical Society; 2023.

Fellowships for the Wild
Postgraduate Wilderness Medicine Fellowships

Alexander J. Axtell, MPAS, PA-C, FAWM[a,b,*]

KEYWORDS

- Wilderness medicine • Medical fellowship • Medical education • APP fellowship

KEY POINTS

- Fellowships are a great way to increase knowledge in a particular specialty
- Wilderness medicine is a new, but growing area of interest
- Fellowship provides 1 year of formal training in wilderness medicine, while the majority of programs are for physician candidates there are opportunities for PA/NP candidates as well

INTRODUCTION

As a new physician assistant (PA), I was interested in finding ways to incorporate my medical work into my love for outdoor activities. The term *"wilderness medicine"* was unknown to me. I tried to be involved in outdoor medical activities but it was difficult while practicing full-time internal medicine. I attended several of the Wilderness Medical Society (WMS) conferences and by chance attended a lecture by Dr Stephanie Lareau. She is currently the program director for a wilderness medicine fellowship at Carilion Clinic in Virginia that accepts both PAs and nurse practitioner (NP).[1] I had been searching for such a program and applied immediately. Within 2 months, I had interviewed with the Virginia tech group, accepted a position as an upcoming fellow and put my notice in with my job in Michigan. I am not known for being a spontaneous person but this decision just felt right, and so far, it has been even better than I expected. There may be others of you out there who have been looking for ways to get involved with wilderness medicine, and hopefully, this article can help you to decide and get a better understanding of what all is involved with a formal wilderness medicine fellowship.

WHAT IS WILDERNESS MEDICINE?

This is probably the most frequently asked question, both before and after the Wilderness fellowship. Wilderness medicine is medical care provided in an austere

a Emergency Medicine, Carilion Clinic, Roanoke, VA, USA; b Virginia Tech Carilion
* 1906 Belleview Avenue SE, Roanoke, VA 24014.
E-mail address: ajaxtell@carilionclinic.org

Physician Assist Clin 9 (2024) 261–264
https://doi.org/10.1016/j.cpha.2023.08.008
2405-7991/24/© 2023 Elsevier Inc. All rights reserved.

environment.[2] Any site where you are outside a formal medical setting can be included in this definition. The most widely accepted time measure of austere is 1 hour away from traditional medical care. Wilderness medicine also puts an emphasis on improvisation and adaptation. Due to the remote nature, decisions regarding what and how much equipment to bring must be carefully considered. The ability to use one piece of equipment/gear for multiple roles or inventing new purposes all together is sometimes necessary. This can be as unusual as repurposing a spare bike tube (on a long-distance bike packing trip) as a sling for an injured arm or as common as a shirt to stabilize a shoulder injury.

A unique aspect of wilderness medicine is the consideration of the environmental effects on your patient and/or rescuers. Within 4 walls, we are seeing patients in a comfortable 68°F room with fluorescent lighting. In contrast, wilderness medicine will involve assessing a patient outdoors, usually with poor or no lighting. Thus, even in moderate temperatures, there is concern for hypothermia if patients and/or rescuers are wet or on the ground for extended periods.

Treatment in an austere setting will also commonly involve some degree of evacuation or transport for a patient. This may involve the need to construct a makeshift litter and rotating rescuers to carry a full-grown adult over perilous terrain. It may even involve clearing a landing area for helicopter evacuation.

Wilderness medicine is a team sport, with practitioners working alongside emergency medical technician (EMT), paramedics, and technical rescue teams. These teams may specialize in swift water rescue, high-angle or low-angle rope rigging, underwater evidence recovery, or cave rescue. Although the wilderness medicine practitioners will not always be an active member of these technical outfits, they need to be familiar with these skills. A wilderness fellowship will typically provide opportunities for certifications in diverse rescues. Wilderness medicine teaches skills and techniques not found in the standard classroom.

APPLYING FOR FELLOWSHIP

Currently, there are 17 WMS-approved fellowships but only 2 accept PA and/or NP applicants, Virginia Tech Carilion and Medical College of Georgia. Although these are non-Accreditation Council for Graduate Medical Education approved fellowships, they still provide rigorous training and experiential learning in wilderness medicine topics. Physician candidates must have completed residency before applying. Although most of the physician applicants are from emergency medicine backgrounds, there is a small but growing number of internal medicine and even family medicine fellows. PA and NP candidates must have a minimum of 2 years work experience.

Having an extensive background in outdoor experience is not necessary. However, most applicants have some experience with outdoor activities including camping, hiking, skiing (water and/or snow), scuba diving, and/or military experience. Applicants may even be an expert in a specific discipline but are looking to expand their knowledge and skill set. It is rare for an applicant to have no outdoor experience because most who are drawn to the specialty are outdoor enthusiasts.

The wilderness medicine fellowships are now part of the residency match program.[3] Although physicians are familiar with the match process, many PA and NP applicants may not be. An applicant must register for the match and rank their desired fellowship programs in the order of preference. This preference order will be based on both research regarding the program and impressions obtained when interviewing at the program. The fellowship programs also rank candidates in the order of their preference for potential fellows. The fellowship and the candidate rankings are submitted to the WMS and candidates are matched to programs based on how they ranked each other. The results of the match are considered binding and are posted on the same "*match*" day for all participants and programs. With only 2 programs that accept PA and NP applicants, the choice of ranking programs is typically much simpler than for a physician applicant. The link to register for the match can be found on the WMS website.[4]

WHAT DOES A WILDERNESS MEDICINE FELLOWSHIP ENTAIL?

A wilderness medicine fellowship can be some of the most fun and fulfilling years of your professional life. It will provide exposure to many different aspects of outdoor recreation and unique medical skills you cannot likely achieve on your own. Although the description is somewhat vague, it is because wilderness medicine fellowship programs are not all the same. The beliefs and background of the program directors differ as does the physical location of the fellowship. The WMS has developed a core curriculum of topics that are part of the fellowship.[5] The "central tenets" of wilderness medicine require an understanding of hypothermia, altitude medicine, frostbite, heat injuries, both marine and land envenomation, disease transmission, medical kit considerations, immunizations, and wilderness evacuation. Although these guidelines act as a blueprint for the fellowship, the implementation is up to the program. The WMS continues to provide peer-reviewed, research-based updates. Although reading the WMS guidelines regarding drowning can be helpful, taking a wilderness lifeguarding course or training in swift water rescue during a 5-day white water rafting trip will help cement these principles. Attending a journal club while eating lunch on the banks of the New River in the newest National Park is a great way to learn.

Each fellowship program has a different variety of teaching styles and will sometimes have a particular focus that can be ascertained during interviews. The Virginia Tech Carilion wilderness fellowship program, for example, has a strong focus on education. The Virginia Tech wilderness fellows are responsible for teaching wilderness first aid to local mountain biking coaches and participating in emergency medical service (EMS)/law-enforcement training events for local and federal agencies. The teaching outreach allows the fellow to become a better instructor. It is important to learn the unique opportunities of each program before joining the match.

When evaluating a program, consider the clinical obligations, the salary, and about funding that is available. While in a wilderness fellowship, there is a clinical requirement to the hospital system of between a 0.4 and 0.6 full-time equivalent position. This typically will be in the emergency department or urgent care center. Specific details will vary per program. It is important to have a strong interest in wilderness medicine but also, one needs to be a strong clinician.

CAREERS IN WILDERNESS MEDICINE

Wilderness fellows, on graduation, have an unlimited number of possibilities. The professional connections made during a fellowship are invaluable. The wilderness medicine world is welcoming but small. Various fellowships work together on journal clubs, conferences, or coauthor articles. This collaboration allows an introduction to others, which can lead to unique opportunities. Previous fellows have attended military courses in mountain medicine not typically open to civilians and have collaborated with leading world experts on reptile envenomation and with the curator of the largest collection of antivenoms in the United States. They have developed training connections and events with national park rangers.

The hard truth is that very few practitioners will make a living solely in wilderness medicine. Most practitioners will have a regular job in a hospital or clinic and participate part time in wilderness medicine activities, paid or volunteer. Many fellows become a medical director for an EMS group or park service. Volunteering with a search and rescue group can also lead to a formal position as medical or safety officer. Working in wilderness medicine requires creativity and persistence to open new opportunities.

During fellowship, there may be opportunities for different specialized certifications. These can range from swift water rescue, scuba instructor, ski patrol, and mountaineering courses including the Diploma in Mountain Medicine. This diploma allows the fellow to become an instructor and can provide opportunities for teaching after graduating from fellowship. Some previous fellows have parlayed conference teaching into free conference registration or travel costs or lodging fees. The very talented teachers have even expanded into a lucrative career of instruction.

SUMMARY

Wilderness medicine is a unique branch of medicine, and a formal fellowship is one of the best ways to expand your understanding and practice. The WMS provides conferences and continuing medical education (CME) events throughout the year. These conferences can be a great place to "*dip your toes*" into the world of wilderness medicine. Further education can include a formal fellowship, with 2 programs accepting PAs and NPs. A fellowship may be fun but it is also a formal year of education and entails the hard work and long hours as with any fellowship. You will be challenged but the skills learned and connections made is worth it.

DISCLOSURE

Current faculty member with Virginia Tech Carilion Wilderness Medicine Fellowship. Received no compensation for my work or from any entities mentioned in article.

REFERENCES

1. Wilderness Medicine NP & PA fellowship. Carilion Clinic. Available at: https://www.carilionclinic.org/gme/wilderness-medicine-np-pa-fellowship#about.   Accessed July 30, 2023.
2. Sward DG, Bennett BL. Wilderness medicine. World J Emerg Med 2014;5(1):5–15. https://doi.org/10.5847/wjem.j.issn.1920-8642.2014.01.001.
3. Davis CA, Lareau S, Haston T, et al. Implementation of a Specialty Society–Sponsored Wilderness Medicine Fellowship Match. Wilderness Environ Med 2023; 34(1):72–6. https://doi.org/10.1016/j.wem.2022.10.007.
4. GME Fellowship Overview. wms.org https://wms.org/WMS/WMS/Learn/GME/GME-Fellowship-Overview.aspx?hkey=3e3f7d9b-b8d8-4a73-8f36-1830fbc826ce.   Accessed March 31, 2023.
5. Lipman GS, Weichenthal L, Stuart Harris N, et al. Core content for wilderness medicine fellowship training of emergency medicine graduates. Acad Emerg Med 2014;21(2):204–7. https://doi.org/10.1111/acem.12304.

Wilderness Medicine Access

Developing Wilderness Medicine Training and Practice Opportunities

Linda Laskowski-Jones, MS, APRN, ACNS-BC, CEN, NEA-BC, FAWM[a,b,c,]*

KEYWORDS

- Wilderness medicine • Training • Practice • Education • Instructor • Moulage
- Low fidelity simulation

KEY POINTS

- Providing wilderness medicine training requires knowledge, preparation, and experience.
- Creating realistic wilderness medicine scenarios promotes participant critical thinking and problem solving in simulated situations.
- Immersive experiences in austere environments enable wilderness medicine enthusiasts to learn and potentially apply their skills in a real-world situation.

INTRODUCTION

Wilderness medicine (WM) education programs offer interdisciplinary health care professionals new knowledge, training, and opportunities that can expand their professional horizons; at the very least, they provide an interesting and novel way to achieve continuing medical education (CME) credit.[1,2] Participants attend these programs for their unique content not generally taught in traditional medical education curricula. Many seek to attain a greater sense of confidence when venturing into outdoor, austere, and wilderness settings, or others look simply to enhance their personal preparedness and meet people who share similar interests.[2]

Even populous areas with ample resources that are typically not considered austere may rapidly become so in the aftermath of natural and man-made disasters. For this reason, WM training offers key knowledge and skills to better perform and maintain safety in the austerity of humanitarian aid in disaster settings and in overall global health work.[3,4] Emerging areas of WM practice that offer new training opportunities include wilderness telemedicine and aerospace medicine.[5,6] WM education and training can be beneficial personally, as a member of the broader community, or as a medical professional deployed on a disaster medical team.

a Appalachian Center for Wilderness Medicine; b Blue Mountain Ski Patrol, Palmerton, PA, USA; c Wolters Kluwer, Philadelphia, PA, USA
* Appalachian Center for Wilderness Medicine, PO Box 2292, Morganton, NC 28680-2292
E-mail address: LindaLJ2622@comcast.net

Physician Assist Clin 9 (2024) 265–277
https://doi.org/10.1016/j.cpha.2023.08.005
2405-7991/24/© 2023 Elsevier Inc. All rights reserved.

Although there are well recognized and standardized continuing education courses available (ie, Advanced Wilderness Life Support [AWLS]), WM education and training takes numerous forms in a wide variety of settings for health care professionals and laypersons covering the full range of WM practice environments. WM content may be offered as part of a physician assistant (PA) or doctor of medicine/doctor of osteopathic medicine residency program curricula, particularly in emergency medicine specialties. It can attract an interdisciplinary audience[7] and can be incorporated into multiple settings including medical conferences, nursing continuing education, PA programs, student wilderness medicine special interest group activities, emergency medical services (EMSs) personnel training, or community venues for the lay public. Interest in learning about this type of practice area has garnered considerable interdisciplinary attention since the (WMS) was established in1982, particularly with the growth of the outdoor and adventure travel industry.[8,9] Being introduced to WM may spark a passion that provides new and ongoing options to learn, educate, practice, and travel.[10] In this author's experience, clinicians attend WM education and training events because they offer a significantly different experience from their usual day-to-day practice settings and role functions; some even see it as a potential path to a fulfilling new career in an austere setting and engaging in a field that they enjoy.

DEVELOPING AND TEACHING WILDERNESS MEDICINE PROGRAMS

WM instructors come from a wide variety of health care backgrounds and experience levels. Some are relatively new to the field, but desire to teach. Teaching others enables WM instructors to further develop their personal level of knowledge and expertise through precourse preparation. Donelan validates this concept by emphasizing that instructors should research the topic they will teach, teach it to themselves, and mentally rehearse it while creating the lesson plan.[11] Teaching offers opportunities to interact with others who have similar interests and may become better connected to WM experts who can serve as teachers and mentors. Taking on an instructor role is a valuable way to advance personal and continuing professional development in WM.

As with any teaching endeavor, the quality of WM training for participants is inextricably linked to the instructor's knowledge, preparation, experience level, and instructional approach with the subject matter. This is best illustrated through the well-known adage in medicine, *see one, do one, teach one*. Each of the components of this adage ultimately relies on the instructor's teaching abilities and effectiveness during the participant's *see one* phase. If the instructor is lacking, what the participant derives from the training will be deficient in quality or even altogether incorrect. Therefore, learners who then *do one* and *teach one* could be propagating misinformation.

Taking stock of personal readiness to competently teach a topic and being able to realistically address any gaps before teaching the subject are essential. Instructors who can relate their own real-world experiences and share WM case anecdotes to clarify or augment the content may promote greater learning, critical thinking, and reasoning abilities through storytelling.[12]

Instructors who develop their own WM presentations should deliver content based on the most recent and best available professional sources. Similar to most health care specialty areas, the field of WM continues to develop consensus-driven and evidence-based practice guidelines (PGs) that arise from the growing body of domestic and international peer-reviewed WM research.[13] The most updated version of the relevant WM PGs should be the foundation of any content taught. However, if an instructor does decide to veer from established, consensus-driven guidelines in a specific situation, that deviation should be made clear to participants along with appropriate and well-reasoned rationale. Perhaps new and compelling information is now available that did not exist when the previous guideline was published, or there are extenuating circumstances not addressed in the PG. Because not all areas of WM are associated with relevant PGs at this time, the most recent peer-reviewed, professional sources should be the basis for educational content. Otherwise, expert opinion is the default.

Teaching Qualifications for Wilderness Medicine Programming

Teaching qualifications vary according to the type of WM content to be taught. Different WM-related organizations that offer standardized and customized courses have their own specific requirements. A simple Internet search using the term "wilderness medicine instructor" yields a vast number of groups offering WM instructor training and teaching opportunities, as well as specific qualifications to teach their courses. However, WM education is also commonly provided in a variety of less formal venues outside of standardized programs, from grand rounds and conferences to online options and onsite practical skills sessions in outdoor environments. Instructors who can relate their own real-world experience and share WM case anecdotes to clarify or augment the content being taught may promote greater learning and reasoning abilities through storytelling.[12]

WILDERNESS MEDICINE TRAINING MODALITIES
Lecture

A lecture format is a common way to teach WM content. Lectures are used in standardized training programs, ie, AWLS, and provide instructor-developed content. Giving a presentation on a WM topic at a hospital in-service, grand rounds, in-person or online conference, or for a community group or organization is an excellent way to introduce the field of WM to those unfamiliar with the specialty. This can also include continuing education to those already experienced in WM. Lectures delivered virtually as a webinar expand both the potential attendee and speaker pools.[14] Audience members with limited or no familiarity with WM may be intrigued enough after exposure to WM content to actively seek additional training options and learn more.[10] Lectures can be excellent vehicles to introduce WM and inspire new WM enthusiasts to bring their varied backgrounds and talents to the field.

Audiovisuals (AVs), such as digital slides with key points and images, can enhance learning and make it more interesting if they are designed well and seamlessly integrated into the presentation (**Fig. 1**).

A caveat, however, is that if the presenter is poorly organized in relation to the AV order, or if the slides contain too much information or are unreadable, the lecturer will likely not achieve the desired results and leave learners frustrated.

Successfully delivering impactful lectures hinges on presenter preparation and well-designed AV materials. Digital slides are ideally prepared on a template with easily discernible colors so that words and images are not obscured by the template background colors or embedded designs. Using a dark print color against a light slide background improves readability.[14] It is best to steer clear of using red and green colors on slides out of consideration for audience members who are colorblind.[14] Word slides are best formatted in a clear font such as Arial and a larger font size (ideally 32 pt or greater.).[14] When creating slides, keep the saying, *less is more* firmly in mind. Slides that contain too much information may be tempting as a speaker aid but are typically unreadable for the audience because they often contain small fonts and are filled with unnecessary wording or graphs that are indiscernible. It is

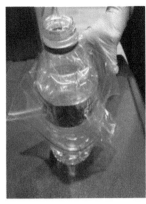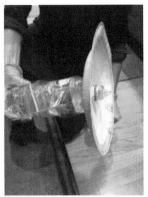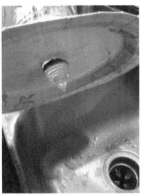

Fig. 1. Improvised wound Irrigation. (Image courtesy Linda Laskowski-Jones.)

challenging for attendees to read a large amount of dense information on a slide while remaining attuned to a lecture.

Keep wording on slides to a minimum and incorporate related images whenever possible to illustrate important concepts. Avoid reading directly from the slides. Know the content. Use the slides to augment lecture delivery, and as a speaker, prompt for the content to be discussed. Consider that each slide requires at least 1 to 2 minutes of lecture time or more. Therefore, a good rule of thumb is that a 60-minute presentation that leaves time for questions and answers should have no more than 25 to 50 slides. Fewer than 25 slides may be necessary if discussion on some slides will be lengthy.

Practical Skills/Psychomotor Learning

Hands-on practice offers participants the opportunity to see and learn how to physically perform new skills in a supervised, controlled, teaching/learning setting. Some participants gravitate toward this type of educational experience and will likely be the first ones volunteering to perform the new skill. Others, however, prefer to remain in the periphery and watch. As WM practice involves both cognitive and psychomotor domains, instructors should assure that everyone is invited and encouraged to perform the skills to gain competence and confidence but must realize that not all will do so. Direct, hands-on participation by everyone in the class is an expectation to successfully complete standardized courses like AWLS but is often unrealistic in many other types of programming (**Fig. 2**).

One of the unique aspects of WM is teaching course participants how to use improvised materials when caring for people in austere environments. Items such as backpacks, sleeping bags, ski poles, canoe or kayak paddles, personal flotation devices, and even tree branches can be transformed into stabilization devices, hypothermia wraps, limb splints, stretchers for movement and evacuation, or shelter materials. Shirts can become arm slings. Envisioning the many possibilities for the alternative uses of items in the WM provider's immediate surroundings requires creativity and practice (**Fig. 3**).

This ability is foundational to WM and enables WM providers to be able to effectively temporize as necessary when managing injuries or illnesses in austere environments outside of well-equipped clinical settings.

It is a good idea for individuals who plan to instruct improvised skill sessions to assemble equipment before teaching the skill session and practice different approaches to using it. One strategy is to dedicate a large duffel bag as a repository

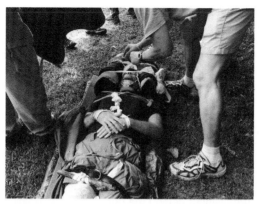

Fig. 2. Class setting up transport of wounded patient. (Image courtesy Linda Laskowski-Jones.)

for storing old, used camping, backpacking, or boating equipment that the owner(s) do not intend to use again in the future. This bag can be tagged or marked for WM training only and taken to various WM educational events to teach hands-on skills using improvised equipment for patient care.

Use of Scenario-Based Teaching

Another aspect of WM training is scenario-based approaches to promote critical thinking and problem solving. It is a strategy that enables participants to combine their

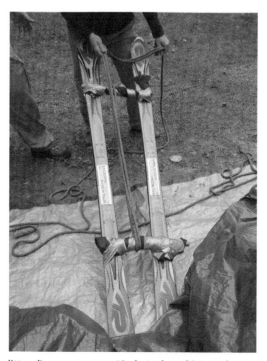

Fig. 3. Skis used as litter. (Image courtesy Linda Laskowski-Jones.)

cognitive knowledge, hands-on skills, and decision-making abilities and apply them directly to manage a "human actor" who role-plays an ill or injured patient in various types of austere environments. Moulage, the practice of using stage make-up, imitation blood, and other items that simulate or mimic wounds, fractures, and amputations, is often brought into scenarios to lend realism by providing visual and tactile cues.[15] These props can often be purchased in stores that sell Halloween costumes and supplies (**Fig. 4**).

A fishing tackle box can help to keep the stage make-up and fake wounds organized. Larger items, such as fake amputated limbs and other body parts can be stored in small duffel bags (**Fig. 5**).

Fake amputated limbs can be placed somewhere in the vicinity of the patient. Then have the participant manage the amputation as well as the amputated body part; body parts must be preserved wrapped in gauze and placed in a plastic bag that is submerged in an ice slurry without getting the body part wet. Training for these actions improve the chances for successful reimplantation.

Creative, home-made props can also be effective in enabling emergency skill performance alongside human actors who respond or are made-up in ways appropriate to the scenarios.[16] An innovative low-fidelity simulator can be easily created using clinical or household items such as nebulizer tubing (for a trachea), gauze, tape, ping pong balls for eyeballs, ribs from the grocery store, ketchup, fake blood, and potatoes.[16] Small potatoes can be great eyeballs used to simulate eye injuries. They can be placed under clothing to simulate the presence of a foreign body or even cut to create a particular deformity. The possibilities are only limited by the instructor's imagination. Banana skins or chicken breasts, for instance, make very good low-fidelity simulators for teaching and practicing suturing skills.

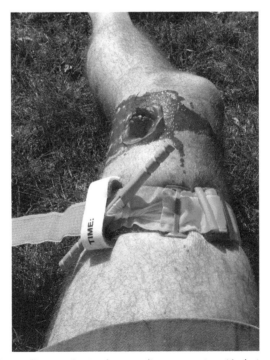

Fig. 4. Moulage 'wound' on patient volunteer. (Image courtesy Linda Laskowski-Jones.)

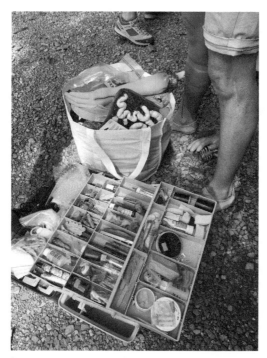

Fig. 5. Tackle box of equipment and bag of limbs. (Image courtesy Linda Laskowski-Jones.)

Narrative WM scenarios can be selected from preexisting course resources or developed by the instructor for the training exercise. The scenarios provide a narrative description of the situation and environment pertinent to the simulated injured or ill person. They include personal details, personal characteristics, medical history (perhaps an anaphylaxis reaction to bee stings or diabetes). The scenarios also provide information about the person's location, including the terrain, climate, weather conditions, and time of day. They may specify how many people are in the ill or injured person's party and how many WM providers are available to assist. Although scenario-based education can be held indoors on a carpeted floor, for example, it is best conducted in realistic, outdoor settings whenever possible.

These scenarios can be planned to offer participants opportunities to learn by working with diverse teams. Although diverse teams are commonplace in health care today, the difference is that in health care facilities, the staff involved in patient care has a health care background. In a wilderness environment, the WM provider's team might be comprised of lay people, ie, a boy scout, an accountant, and/or a carpenter, who happen to be in the area and willing to help. The WM provider must then decide what types of skills can be delegated or taught to these people so that they can be assets in the patient care and evacuation effort.

These types of scenarios can also involve a group of course participants working together to accomplish group problem-solving. The instructors can facilitate their work by injecting key findings as the simulated patient is evaluated and ask thought-provoking questions about various group decisions. After the scenario ends, the instructors can host a debriefing session to elicit feedback, provide relevant observations, offer an overall critique, and suggest various alternative management options. This is also the time to address any participant questions or lingering concerns. Techniques to engage class participants as well as debriefing after the scenarios conclude are considered essential to effective simulations.[15]

Fellowships

Fellowship programs in WM are available and are offered in different formats.

1. The WMS awards the Fellowship in the Academy of Wilderness Medicine upon successful program completion.[17] The interdisciplinary program entails completing a formalized WM course curriculum including a required number of core and elective CME credits and experience credits.
2. A growing number of hospitals and health care organizations offer WM fellowship programs.[18] This type of WM fellowship program typically consists of 1 to 2 years of focused WM education and hands-on skills. As of 2023, the small number of hospital-based WM fellowship programs are primarily available for physicians in emergency medicine and family practice; however, there are 2 US-based WM fellowship for nurse practitioners (NPs) and PAs that is embedded within the Physician WM fellowship (https://www.carilionclinic.org/gme/wilderness-medicine-np-pa-fellowship#about).[18,19] These WM fellowships offer a salary and consist of a postgraduate WM training curriculum and practical experiences in WM, in addition to a requirement to work assigned hospital shifts. Little consistency has been identified in the curricula between the different fellowship programs, although specific recommendations exist in the literature for implementing a standardized WM curriculum with core content.[18,20] Because WM is a team sport, this author strongly supports making these types of programs more widely available to PAs and NPs.

WILDERNESS MEDICINE PRACTICE OPPORTUNITIES

Ways to both stimulate interest in WM as well as give WM enthusiasts practice opportunities include arranging time to gain observational, hands-on, and immersive experiences with seasoned WM providers in a wide range of practice settings. Whether or not WM enthusiasts can observe or apply their skills with patients in these settings is based on both professional licensure laws and the policies of the organizations providing the practical experience. It is important to investigate the licensure requirements and regulations prior to embarking on such an opportunity. Assure that professional liability coverage will be uninterrupted during the WM experience, and arrange for any necessary provisions to be added to the policy as needed.

Selected Observational and Hands-on Practice Options

Some of the best observational and hands-on experiences entail spending time with WM providers in situations that offer frequent patient encounters involving problems and management strategies in the WM domain. The availability of these experiences in some locations, such as urban environments, may be quite limited, but they are still possible through medical partnerships with outdoor industries, participation on disaster teams, medical skills training, and EMS operations.[9,21] Travel to a more remote location to meet the WM enthusiasts' goals may become necessary and, of course, that depends on participants' ability and willingness to travel.

Volunteer Work at Wilderness Medicine Events

A widely available option for gaining WM practical experience is to serve as a volunteer on event medical teams for triathlons, marathons, ultramarathons, and other types of adventure races.[22] These races are held throughout the United States and abroad, even in some urban areas (eg, the Chicago Marathon) and may attract a large number of competitors and spectators. Adventure races include mud runs and obstacle races held at ski areas, state and national parks, or in remote natural areas.[23] Endurance races and ultramarathons are often held in mountain and desert environments; the terrain can be extreme.[23] Some adventure races are stage races or multiday events with competitors pushing their physical and psychological limits.[22] Event medical volunteers will see the impact of weather conditions on participants, as well as the range of physiologic derangements, illnesses, and injuries that can occur.[23] WM skills may become necessary due to limited medical resources and the lack of the usual clinical infrastructure of the emergency department, as well as the potential difficulties in patient evacuation when terrain is challenging.[22,23]

Work with Search and Rescue Teams

Another WM practical experience option is to connect with a search and rescue (SAR) team and seek permission to attend one or more of their meetings, training sessions, and even potential deployments or "call-outs."[24] Some SAR teams are very busy with call-outs several times a week. SAR teams that provide their services to state and national parks or natural areas that attract a high volume of visitors or cover mountainous areas with popular hiking or climbing routes fall into this category. The level of the WM enthusiast's mountaineering skills and outdoor experience will likely determine the type and degree of participation that is allowed with the SAR team, if the team has policies that allow a limited number of observers. With that said, there are many aspects of the SAR response, including the command post operations, that provide coordination and logistical support. Observational experiences with these aspects of SAR can be beneficial to learners who have no background or previous exposure to SAR. Overall, the SAR experience in remote or wilderness environments introduces the challenges, skills, training, and operations that give observers new knowledge and insights into this critically important service to outdoor enthusiasts.[24]

Remote Clinical Settings

Remote clinical settings offer another option for getting practical experience through organizations providing medical volunteerism opportunities and potentially, paid positions, if available. These include critical access hospitals, medical clinics, and outposts that serve rural locations, national parks, wilderness areas, and other highly austere environments on a global scale. These locales typically have a greater number of human-wild animal encounters, toxic plant exposures, venomous bites and stings, insect-borne disease, water-borne pathogens, and environmental issues (ie, extremes of heat, cold, wet conditions, and lightning). In addition to gaining insights into managing these conditions, clinicians in remote health care settings will acquire a greater appreciation for the challenges of treating patients in resource-limited environments, as well as realize the impact of weather on patient evacuation if a higher level of care is needed. Health care professionals who seek this type of experiences must have adequate WM training before practicing in these environments.[3] An example of an extreme, remote outpost is the medical tent located at Mount Everest Base Camp where medical volunteers serve as the health care providers during the climbing season. Aerospace settings are also considered extreme environments that offer new opportunities for WM knowledge, skills, and practice.[6]

Ski Patrols

Members of ski patrols perform emergency care for those injured while participating in snow sports: skiing, snowboarding, and snow tubing. Many patrols now engage in emergency care coverage for summertime activities held at ski areas and resorts:

mountain biking, ropes courses, and hiking. They also respond to care for ill or injured persons on the premises. Most ski patrols use improvised techniques as part of their training and management of patients. They work in all manner of weather conditions, from severe cold, heavy snow, and high wind to moderate temperatures, wet weather, and ice. They assess and mitigate avalanche risk and identify and address other potential safety issues for patrons and mountain personnel. Their functions include SAR, mountaineering, and lift evacuation procedures if the ski lift should cease to be functional.

For those with snow sport skills, a ski patrol management-approved "ride along" or observation experience with the ski patrol offers an excellent WM learning opportunity. Participants in this setting will don their skis or snowboard to gain a greater understanding of working in cold weather conditions, cold-induced injuries, seasonal ski patrol operations, and special techniques. Participants will see the improvised, temporized management of musculoskeletal trauma on the mountain, as well as management strategies for other types of injuries and illnesses that may occur at the ski area. If the WM participant is not a snow sport aficionado or desires an alternative indoor experience, working with ski patrol or other health care professionals in the aid room or associated medical clinic may be an option.

Immersive Experiences

Immersive experiences enable health care professionals to provide hands-on care to persons who require medical management. These types of experiences might involve days to weeks or more in the WM practice environment. These experiences can be associated with organizations that hold large group gatherings in outdoor settings and hire experienced, licensed health care providers to manage participants' injuries or health conditions. Examples include the medical team for the annual National Scout jamboree or camps affiliated with a wide variety of groups that host outdoor events and activities for youth and adults.

Other immersive experiences involve volunteer expeditions and humanitarian or disaster aid work in austere settings.[25] WM skills, including water purification techniques and knowledge of the local flora, fauna, and pathogens, are an asset in these settings. Those who deploy are best advised to go with organizations and health care providers that are well experienced in this type of work. Not only are there profound resource limitations in settings that require disaster or humanitarian aid as well as special cultural considerations, but there are also significant personal safety risks to the WM provider that must be mitigated to the greatest degree possible.[4,26] If the provider is planning to leave the United States for this type of service experience, reviewing governmental advisories, including the Center for Disease Control website, to learn about security risks, endemic diseases, and recommendations for prophylaxis and treatment is essential. A travel medicine specialist should be consulted to provide the required or recommended vaccines over a period that allows them to take effect before trip departure. The travel medicine specialist can also offer other advice that can help travelers maintain personal wellness and safety.

Depending on the location of travel and the humanitarian aid objective, the WM provider is likely to encounter health disorders rarely seen in the United States, such as malaria, human botfly infestations, and human rabies. These disorders, as well as many others, fall into the WM knowledge domain. These are excellent opportunities to expand the WM provider's repertoire of experiences outside of the four walls of traditional medical facilities.[4]

Deploying as a volunteer medical aid worker in a disaster situation also enables opportunities for hands-on WM practice. However, it involves a greater degree of risk and requires greater diligence and pre-travel preparation. Though the nature and extent of the disaster can include urban areas, the resulting resource limitations can transform an otherwise resource-rich landscape into an austere environment. Widespread theft and violence are possible when stable societal structures and resources are disrupted. It is best to deploy with a team of experienced disaster medical professionals or a disaster aid organization skilled in providing medical care in disaster settings, rather than deciding to self-deploy alone into a dangerous, uncontrolled situation.[27]

Disaster medical workers must have the required up-to-date vaccines pertinent to the travel destination and enough personal supplies to meet medication, clothing, shelter, food, and fluid needs, potentially for the duration of the deployment. Deciding to deploy also comes down to taking stock of personal medical needs and if they could impact individual safety on a disaster deployment, including if that risk can be mitigated. This is a critical decision-making point; it is always best to avoid becoming a casualty that might divert medical attention away from those directly impacted by the disaster. If the decision is to go with a disaster medical group, remain alert to all risks common to that specific area of the world: floodwaters with raw sewage, poisonous snakes, electric hazards, food-borne and/or water-borne pathogens, and unstable structures. Those impacted may have lost access to required medications and have exacerbations of diseases and disorders as well as many different degrees of trauma. Improvised techniques may be necessary for patient evacuation and care.[27]

SUMMARY

Teaching medical professionals through creative, dynamic, and enjoyable ways helps to inspire knowledge and creativity, as well as prepares health care professionals to practice in unique settings. This is an overview of success strategies and options to train and provide practical experiences for health care professionals who desire to pursue WM education. Because WM is a team sport with a strong interdisciplinary component, it is helpful to train with a variety of clinicians and even nonclinicians who have wilderness experience. These can include survival experts, cartographers, park rangers, botanists, herpetologists, marine biologists, and/or environmental experts along with others. The field is a fascinating one that offers nearly unlimited personal and professional growth potential. The options described represent only a sampling of the many possible approaches to WM education and fieldwork.

DISCLOSURES

The author warrants that this article is original and has not been submitted to any other publication for consideration. The author has no commercial or financial conflicts of interest related to the contents of this article, nor have received any funding sources for this scholarly work. The author is the Editor-in-Chief of *Nursing* (Nursing) for Wolters Kluwer.

REFERENCES

1. Stuart CM, Tindle KC, Phillips LL. Characteristics and Motivating Factors of Attendees of a Regional Student-Run Wilderness Medicine Conference. Wilderness Environ Med 2019;30(4):461–7.
2. Trierweiler RW. The Who and Why of Wilderness Medicine Conference Attendance. Wilderness Environ Med 2013;24(1):84.
3. Lemery J, Sacco D, Kulkarni A, et al. Wilderness medicine within global health: a strategy for less risk and more reward. Wilderness Environ Med 2012;23(1):84–8.

4. Matthew J. The role of wilderness medicine training in resource-limited settings. Afr J Emerg Med 2016;6(4):172–3.
5. Davis CB, Lorentzen AK, Patel H, et al. The Intersection of Telemedicine and Wilderness Care: Past, Present, and Future. Wilderness Environ Med 2022;33(2):224–31.
6. Babu G, Upchurch BD, Young WH, et al. Medicine in Extreme Environments: A New Medical Student Elective Class for Wilderness, Aerospace, Hyperbaric, Exercise, and Combat Medicine. Wilderness Environ Med 2020;31(1):110–5.
7. Lareau SA, Robinson PE, Wentworth SS, et al. Impact of a student-organized conference on wilderness medicine education. Wilderness Environ Med 2014;25(1):120–1.
8. Bowman WD. Wilderness Medical Society: The First Dozen Years. J Wilderness Med 1994;5(3):237–47.
9. Donelan S. Introduction to 'Wilderness medicine education in the city: a new paradigm'. Wilderness Environ Med 2008;19(3):205.
10. Belyea A, Fish A, Phillips L. Wilderness Medicine Physician Education: How an Elective Can Spark a Fire. Cureus 2021;13(5):e15317.
11. Donelan S. Secrets of a Successful Lecture. Wilderness Environ Med 1999;10(3):185–8.
12. Winkelman C, Kelley C, Savrin C. Case histories in the education of advanced practice nurses. Crit Care Nurse 2012;32(4):e1–17.
13. Sward DG, Bennett BL. Wilderness medicine. World J Emerg Med 2014;5(1):5–15.
14. Topor DR, Budson AE. Twelve tips to present an effective webinar. Med Teach 2020;42(11):1216–20.
15. Stokes-Parish JB, Duvivier R, Jolly B. Investigating the impact of moulage on simulation engagement - A systematic review. Nurse Educ Today 2018;64:49–55.
16. Saxon KD, Kapadia AP, Juneja NS, et al. How to teach emergency procedural skills in an outdoor environment using low-fidelity simulation. Wilderness Environ Med 2014;25(1):50–5.
17. Wilderness Medical Society. FAWM: Fellowship in the Academy of Wilderness Medicine. Available at: https://wms.org/WMS/Get-Certified/FAWM/Home.aspx?hkey=f1152894-904a-4d75-bac2-d0c49f108fe6 . Accessed April 14, 2022.
18. Holstrom-Mercader M, Kass D, Corsetti M, et al. Wilderness Medicine Curricula in United States EMS Fellowship, Emergency Medicine Residency, and Wilderness Medicine Programs. Prehosp Disaster Med 2022;37(6):800–5.
19. Carilion Clinic. Wilderness Medicine NP & PA Fellowship. Available at: https://www.carilionclinic.org/gme/wilderness-medicine-np-pa-fellowship#about Accessed: April 14, 2023.
20. Lipman GS, Weichenthal L, Stuart Harris N, et al. Core content for wilderness medicine fellowship training of emergency medicine graduates. Acad Emerg Med 2014;21(2):204–7.
21. Lemery J, Tedeschi C, Miner T. Wilderness medicine education in the city: a new paradigm. Wilderness Environ Med 2008;19(3):206–9.
22. Joslin J, Mularella J, Schreffler S, et al. Race Medicine: A Novel Educational Experience for GME Learners. Wilderness Environ Med 2015;26(4):576–7.
23. Laskowski-Jones L, Caudell MJ, Hawkins SC, et al. Extreme event medicine: considerations for the organization of out-of-hospital care during obstacle, adventure and endurance competitions. Emerg Med J 2017;34(10):680–5.
24. Larsen J, Blagnys H, Cooper B, et al. Mountain Rescue Casualty Care and the Undergraduate Medical Elective. Wilderness Environ Med 2019;30(2):210–6.

25. Imray CH, Grocott MP, Wilson MH, et al. Extreme, expedition, and wilderness medicine. Lancet 2015;386(10012):2520–5.
26. Panosian C. Courting danger while doing good–protecting global health workers from harm. N Engl J Med 2010;363(26):2484–5.
27. Arnaouti MKC, Cahill G, Baird MD, et al. Medical disaster response: A critical analysis of the 2010 Haiti earthquake. Front Public Health 2022;10:995595. Published 2022 Nov 1.

Medicine on the Trail
Ultramarathon Medical Coverage

Joshua Nichols, MD[a],*, Eric Olsen, PA-C[b], Stephanie Lareau, MD[c]

KEYWORDS

- Ultramarathons • Race medicine • Event medicine • Medical support
- Hyponatremia • Endurance events

KEY POINTS

- Ultramarathoners are at risk for medical conditions ranging from overuse injuries to trauma to cardiac arrest.
- Providing race support requires significant planning and knowledge of common and life-threatening medical conditions in addition to race location and logistics.
- Medical kits should be created to address both serious but uncommon conditions and common but less serious conditions.
- Planning is the key to providing effective medical coverage.

INTRODUCTION

Ultramarathons are long-distance races, defined as any distance over 42.2 km or 26.2 miles. Races often range from 50 to 100 miles with terrain varying from paved roads to remote single-track trails. Races can be loops, out and back, or one-way courses. They are often in remote environments, such as national forests.[1] When preparing to provide medical support for races, there are many unique factors to consider. These range from injury types and patterns to methods to access runners and communications to both the base and the closest support services.

CLINICS CARE POINTS

When providing medical support for endurance running races, the provider should be prepared to care for the following critical medical conditions.

- Sudden Cardiac Death
- Acute Asthma Exacerbation

---

[a] Virginia Tech Carilion School of Medicine, 1906 Belleview Avenue, Roanoke, VA 24014, USA;
[b] Emergency Medicine, Carilion Clinic; [c] Emergency Medicine, Virginia Tech Carilion School of Medicine
* Corresponding author.
E-mail address: jcnichols@carilionclinic.org

Physician Assist Clin 9 (2024) 279–289
https://doi.org/10.1016/j.cpha.2023.08.009
2405-7991/24/© 2023 Elsevier Inc. All rights reserved.

- Anaphylaxis
- Hypoglycemia
- Hyponatremia
- Hypothermia
- Hyperthermia
- Dehydration
- Trauma
- Orthopedic Injuries
- Foot Care
- Endurance Gastroparesis
- Cold Injury
- Corneal Edema

PRE-RACE PREPARATION

Event medical coverage is very variable and unpredictable. Some events, such as the Ironman, have a large team of physicians, nurses, athletic trainers. and paramedics throughout the course with a specified medical tent capable of providing intravenous (IV) fluids, performing electrocardiographies, ultrasounds, and point-of-care (POC) laboratory tests. Other races may just rely on a few volunteers with wilderness first aid training and personal medical kits containing basic first aid materials. When ultramarathon participants were surveyed, 83.2% felt events should provide a minimum level of medical support with first aid and emergency medical transport. Of those who needed medical care during an event, 74% felt medical care was adequate.[2]

When preparing to provide medical support for an event, there are many factors for consideration. Knowing the approximate number of participants helps determine the volume of resources needed. It is important to become familiar with the course and terrain to know if the course is accessible by car, all-terrain vehicle, or only by foot. It is vital to have a map of the course, aid stations, and additional access points when planning assistance. If the event has occurred before, race directors often know of problems spots on the course. Weather and conditions can also play an important role in planning.[1]

One needs to know if there is cell phone service for the whole course or if radio coverage is needed and available. Often a race director has a pre-defined communication plan. Having a pre-defined method for communicating current location or location last seen of an injured athlete is imperative. Global positioning systems (GPS) coordinates are often used; however, new systems like *"What3words"* are becoming more popular with search and rescue. *"What3words"* is an application that will designate 3 words for any location selected (including the current) location within about 3 m. Another user can enter these same words to find the location. This information is easier to relay over radio communications. Depending on the size of the event, notifying local emergency medical services (EMS) and hospitals is prudent. Some events will have local standby EMS on site. This is more common in rural or remote areas where an event with thousands of participants could easily overwhelm a local medical system.

Medical team and team preparedness are important. Prior triathlon literature has suggested that there should be on average 1 physician per 200 athletes and 1 nurse per 100 athletes.[3] As roles are often filled by volunteers, a varied team of wilderness first responders, nurses, medics, physician assistants, nurse practitioners, and physicians can create a successful team for medical care. All medical providers should have training in conditions seen during ultramarathons. Pre-hospital and event medicine experience are useful but not required of every volunteer.

MEDICAL KIT DESIGN BASED ON SERIOUS DISEASE PROCESSES

When designing a medical kit for endurance running race support, it is important to consider both the less common but serious medical conditions and more common but less serious medical conditions likely to be encountered. Equipment for serious medical pathologies likely to be encountered during endurance running race must be available (**Table 1**).

CARDIAC ARREST

A sudden cardiac event can happen anywhere. During long-duration physical activity, such as in ultramarathons or in the race preparation phase, the cardiovascular system is under considerable stress. This can lead to exercise-induced cardiac remodeling often referred to as runner's heart. In endurance athletes, this presents as an enlarged right atrium and right ventricle. This right-sided dilation can lead to arrhythmias causing the runner to experience a sudden collapse with a non-perfusing rhythm.[4]

The runner experiencing a sudden collapse during the event should be assessed quickly for the presence of a pulse. If no pulse is present, initiation of high-quality cardiopulmonary resuscitation(CPR) and application of an automated external defibrillator will greatly increase the chances for a positive outcome. The runner will require transportation to the nearest medical center that can provide appropriate care.[5] It is important to have a mechanism to notify the racer's family, typically a bib number or 'electronic bib tags" linked to racer information. A plan to debrief those involved in the care of a collapsed athlete is imperative for caregivers' psychological well-being.

ASTHMA/BRONCHOSPASM

Runners often suffer from an exercise-induced bronchoconstriction (EIB). EIB can affect those with or without asthma. The general population without asthma has a <20% prevalence of experiencing EIB whereas the endurance athlete with asthma has an occurrence prevalence of 30% to 70%.[6] EIB is thought to be caused by the lung parenchyma becoming hyperosmolar and inducing an inflammatory response after losing heat and moisture to cold, dry air.[7]

Table 1
Suggested supplies and equipment for serious race-related conditions

Pathology	Supplies
Sudden Cardiac Death	AED, cardiac monitor, ACLS medications
Acute Asthma Exacerbation	MDI vs nebulizer w/duo nebs (depending on electricity available); stethoscope, pulse oximeter
Hypoglycemia	Sugary drinks, glucose gel, D5W or D10 W (and IV supplies), intranasal or intramuscular glucagon, POC glucometer
Hyponatremia	Salty drinks, hypertonic fluids; POC laboratory equipment
Trauma	C-collar, splinting supplies, hemostatic gauze, tourniquet, roller gauze, 4 × 4's, elastic wrap, needle decompression with flutter valve, triangle bandage, collapsible liter, 4 × 4 vehicle
Hypothermia	Mylar blanket, insulating blankets, caloric-dense foods/drinks, heat source, thermometer

Abbreviations: AED, automated external defibrillator; ACLS, advanced cardiovascular life support; POC, point of care; MDI, metered dose inhaler; nebs, nebulizer; D5W, dextrose 5% in water; C-collar, cervical collar; 4 × 4s, 4 in by 4 in gauze.

Acute bronchoconstriction and asthma exacerbations can be life-threatening yet usually manageable. Cold air, prolonged exertion, or exposure to a multitude of new environmental allergens can trigger an exacerbation. Typically, athletes will provide a history of asthma or similar symptoms with training. Some runners will carry a rescue inhaler during the event and use it when they feel the characteristic chest tightness associated with bronchospasm. Diagnosis and treatment are complicated when a runner has no history of asthma as the differential diagnosis can include cardiac etiologies, trauma, pulmonary embolism, or infection.

Assessing blood oxygen saturation with a portable pulse oximeter, auscultating for expiratory wheezing, and gauging response to beta agonists can help differentiate among etiologies causing shortness of breath. It is useful to stock metered-dose inhalers or a nebulizer (if in a medical tent) with beta adrenergic agonist and anticholinergic medications.

ANAPHYLAXIS

Although not unique to endurance events, anaphylaxis can affect athletes during races. Anaphylaxis is type 1 hypersensitivity reaction, involving multiple organ systems including integument, respiratory, and/or gastrointestinal (GI) symptoms after ingestion or exposure to an allergen. Allergens that may be commonly encountered during endurance events are Hymenoptera, nuts, and red meats. Anaphylaxis affects between 1.6% and 2% of Americans.[8]

Red meat allergy, also known as the alpha-gal allergy, comes from exposure to tick bites from the Lone Star tick. It creates an allergy to alpha-galactose protein which is found in red meats such as beef and pork. By-products of these mammals can also be found in other food products. As runners spend significant time outdoors in tick-prone areas, this population has a higher risk. Typically, initial exposures result in mild symptoms, a rash, or GI upset, but repeated exposure can lead to full-blown anaphylaxis. Many aid stations have protein snacks such as bacon that could put athletes at risk. Symptoms can be delayed for hours after ingestion of red meat.

Aid stations may also have foods containing nuts which can be dangerous for runners with nut allergies. Being aware of these allergies prior to the race can be helpful when stocking aid stations or creating nut-free zones at aid stations.

The treatment for anaphylaxis is epinephrine, which is a prescription medication most commonly found in an autoinjector or pre-filled syringe. Athletes with known severe allergy or with past anaphylaxis often carry an epinephrine auto injector with them on the course. Epinephrine must be kept in a temperature-stable environment and is less effective after temperature excursions. There is an off-label way to open a used autoinjector to get additional doses which can be useful if a rebound reaction occurs in an austere environment.[9]

Adjunct treatments include histamine blockers such as diphenhydramine (Type 1) and ranitidine (Type 2) as well as the use of steroids. Some patients with a history of reactive airway disease or asthma who present with wheezing may benefit from bronchodilators (often albuterol). Anyone with a severe allergic reaction or anaphylaxis should be evacuated for definitive care, further monitoring and should not continue with the event.

HYPOGLYCEMIA

Hypoglycemia is defined as blood glucose of less than 70 mg/dL. Although hypoglycemia is more commonly a concern among diabetic runners, as exercise can increase insulin sensitivity, it is also seen in non-diabetic runners. During extended periods of physical exertion, the body breaks down glycogen stores which release glucose.

The glucose can then be used for aerobic and anaerobic metabolism used to generate ATP needed for muscle contraction. Muscle glycogen is depleted more rapidly in high-intensity activities such as sprinting, but eventually becomes depleted in endurance events. When muscle and liver glycogen stores are both depleted, the liver performs gluconeogenesis to provide glucose stores to the brain and muscles; however, the rate of production does not meet the rate of demand during exercise. For these reasons, proper nutrition prior to and during endurance events is vital for sufficient glycogen stores to prevent hypoglycemia.[10]

Hypoglycemia typically presents with sweating, irritability, confusion, and difficulty with coordination. Untreated or unrecognized, it can ultimately lead to seizures, coma, and death. Initial treatment for any altered athlete should include rest and simple carbohydrates often glucose-containing gels or tablets. If hypoglycemia is suspected and swallowing is a concern, a small amount of glucose gel can be put inside the buccal mucosa where it will be absorbed. Glucagon, as used in severely altered diabetics, may not be effective as it works to signal the liver to perform glycogenolysis, changing glycogen into useable glucose. This is impossible if liver glycogen stores have already been depleted. In a severely altered or unconscious patient, if available, an intravenous (IV) of 10% dextrose (D10) or 50% dextrose (D50) can be administered via venous or intraosseous access.

EXERCISE-ASSOCIATED HYPONATREMIA

Exercise-associated hyponatremia (EAH) is an insidious pathology. Runners will often stop at multiple drink stations and ingest far more water than needed to adequately address their thirst, thus contributing to a dilutional hyponatremia. The symptoms for EAH are somewhat vague so the diagnosis needs to be in the differential. Runners who have developed hyponatremia, serum sodium less than 135meq/dL, can start to experience nausea, vomiting, and headache in the early stages. When left untreated, progression includes confusion, altered mental status, and seizures.[11]

If caught early and the patient still has an intact gag reflex, salt drinks and salty snacks can be encouraged. If the patient can tolerate oral fluids, 800 mg of sodium in 200 mL of water or 4 bouillon cubes in 125 mL of water is an appropriate oral hypertonic solution. The bouillon cubes could be dissolved in a thermos of hot water or prepared prior to the event.[12] If POC laboratory equipment is available, determining the runner's serum sodium level can direct care. For treatment of patients with symptomatic hyponatremia who are unable to tolerate oral intake, consider administering intravenous hypertonic saline (3% NaCl), 100ml bolus over a 10 minute period. As hypertonic saline can cause issues with pontine demyelination, it is only used when severe neurologic symptoms such as seizures occur. Patients with severe hyponatremia should be evacuated to the nearest capable medical facility. Unlike chronic hyponatremia, rapid correction of acute hyponatremia is important and potentially lifesaving.

HYPOTHERMIA

Cold, wet, windy, or rapidly changing weather patterns can put race participants at risk for hypothermia. Severity of hypothermia will determine treatment.

Hypothermia can be classified as follows:.

- Cold stress
- Mild
- Moderate
- Severe

Runners with cold stress will have a body temperature greater than 95°F. These runners will be conscious and alert with normal movement although they will be shivering. Treatment for these patients consists of reducing heat loss by changing into warm dry clothing, having the patient move around to warm up, and providing high-calorie food or drink. When symptoms have improved, these patients can usually continue racing or assist in their own evacuation.

Mild hypothermia is classified as core body temperature approximately 89.6°F to 95°F. These patients will be conscious and alert but will develop abnormal movement patterns including impaired coordination. They will also be shivering. Treatment for these patients includes active rewarming with an external heat source, providing a vapor barrier and insulation, and providing high-calorie food and drink. These patients should be handled gently and encouraged to sit or lie down while treatment is initiated. If symptoms do not resolve, these patients will need to be evacuated.

Moderate hypothermia is classified as core body temperature between 82.4°F and 89.6°F. These patients are conscious but no longer alert. They have impaired movement and have lost the drive to shiver. These patients should be handled very carefully in order to avoid inducing cardiac arrhythmias. Patients should be kept horizontal and not allowed to stand or walk. A vapor barrier and insulation should be applied and heat applied to the patient's trunk. These patients should not be given oral nutrition due to the risk of aspiration. These patients will need to be evacuated carefully.

Severe hypothermia is classified as a core body temperature less than 82.4°F. These patients are no longer conscious or shivering. These patients should be treated similarly to moderate hypothermia. They should be kept horizontal, and handled carefully to avoid inducing arrhythmia. If no obvious vital signs are present, then an every 60-second pulse and respiration check should be initiated. In severe hypothermia, pulse and breathing rate may be significantly slowed, so it is imperative to check vital signs for a longer period. If no breathing or pulse is present, CPR should be initiated and evacuation should be initiated. Termination of resuscitation efforts should not be considered until the patient is normothermic.[13]

TRAUMA

Trauma can range from sprains, strains, and/or fractures to unprotected falls associated with traumatic arrests. Injuries can occur in difficult to access terrain with a significant delay in reaching the patient. Patients with minor injuries may be able to evacuate under their own power or with the assistance of rescuers, often after receiving treatment. Patients with major injuries may require mobilization and coordination of external EMS resources in order to successfully evacuate.

It is important to consider that the trauma may be secondary to a medical issue. Hypoglycemia or hyponatremia may lead to a fall and the underlying condition will also need to be evaluated and addressed. When caring for an injured or immobilized athlete, efforts must be made to prevent hypothermia. This may include discreetly removing wet or sweaty clothes while protecting privacy and applying a vapor barrier (space blanket or tarp).

MEDICAL KIT DESIGN BASED ON COMMON DISEASE PROCESSES

It is important to include in medical kit planning, disease processes that are more common but less serious (**Table 2**). This will maximize usefulness of the medical team and likely increase satisfaction of participants.

Table 2	
Suggested supplies and equipment for common, minor race-related conditions	
Pathology	**Supplies**
Orthopedic Injuries	Flexible aluminum splints, elastic bandages, padding, athletic tape, over-the-counter (OTC) oral medications such as acetaminophen or ibuprofen, OTC pain relief creams or rubs
Blisters/Foot Care	Paper tape, benzoin, alcohol prep pads, needle, adhesive tape, mole skin, colloid gel, oral antibiotics (cephalexin), dry socks
Gastrointestinal Illness	Ondansetron, metoclopramide, loperamide, electrolyte-containing fluids
Cold Injury	Mylar blanket, wool blankets, hand warmers
Corneal Edema	Eye chart, saline eye drops

ORTHOPEDIC INJURIES

Orthopedic injuries, while not life threatening, are the most common injuries seen in ultramarathon runners. Initial assessment should include a thorough examination of the skin integrity, neurovascular status, and examination of the joint above and below the injury. Any racer with neurovascular compromise, especially due to a displaced joint, should be expeditiously evacuated. Depending on provider training and available resources, reduction could be attempted. It is important to look for signs indicating a fracture as opposed to a sprain or strain. There are validated clinical decision tools, such as the Ottawa ankle and knee rules, that can assist with ruling out fractures.[14] Racers with suspected fractures should not continue in the race. Suspected fractures should be splinted, often using flexible aluminum splints, adequate padding, and elastic bandages. Sprains and strains can also be taped, wrapped, or splinted. For upper extremity injuries, a sling can be helpful. Depending on the degree of injury, some racers may opt to try to continue the race. Over-the-counter pain relief medications such as acetaminophen or ibuprofen can be considered.

BLISTER AND FOOT CARE

Foot care is tremendously important for runners. Blisters have been reported to account for up to 75% of medical care during ultramarathons.[15] Blisters are formed by friction and sheer stress, creating a fluid-filled pocket between the stratum granulosum and spinosum. Wet feet, carrying increased weight, and poorly fitting shoes can increase blister formation. Multiple studies have not demonstrated any one method that significantly prevents blister formation.[16] It is important for the runner to be aware of areas of their feet which are prone to developing hot spots and blisters. The hot spot is a friction point that can develop into a blister if not addressed promptly. Care needs to be taken to reduce the friction by applying a barrier such as paper tape or mole skin.

There is minimal evidence on treating blisters although one prospective study demonstrated draining blisters in the first 24 hours led to quickest healing.[17] Otherwise expert opinion is typically to clean the area with alcohol and puncture the dependent portion of the blister with a needle, to allow the fluid to drain. The blister then should be covered with paper tape, then a benzoin-type adhesive, and finally with adhesive tape. Rounded edges on the adhesive tape tend to help tape stay in place. If blisters have already been deroofed, using a hydrocolloid pad over the base can also help. Clean, dry socks, dry shoes, allowing feet to dry will also help prevent additional damage.[18] Although rare, necrotizing soft tissue infections ultimately leading to amputation has been reported as a complication of blisters in an ultramarathon runner.[19] Early recognition, local wound care, and oral antibiotics should be used for infected blisters. There is some evidence that topical antibiotic ointment can *increase* blister formation, so it should be not used if the runner is continuing in the event.

GASTROINTESTINAL ILLNESS

A significant number of runners will experience GI) symptoms, ranging from relative benign nausea/bloating to more severe ischemic colitis. Runners are also not immune from general GI illnesses (traveler's diarrhea) or more serious conditions (appendicitis).

Exercise-associated gastroparesis, or *Slosh Gut*, is decreased GI motility leading to the sensation of liquids sloshing around within the stomach. This has associated nausea, vomiting, and discomfort. Loss of appetite and loss of desire to drink can occur, leading to nutrition and hydration deficiencies and jeopardizing runners' ability to finish the race. These symptoms can often be managed successfully with anti-nausea medication such as ondansetron or metoclopramide.[20] Small amounts of electrolyte-containing fluids should be encouraged.

Runner's diarrhea is also common occurrence in ultramarathon running. The etiology is thought to be multifactorial including mechanical, nutritional, and ischemic causes. Avoidance of the ingestion of fiber, fat, protein, high-carbohydrate substances, (fermentable oligosaccharides, disaccharides, monosaccharides, and polyols), nonsteroidal anti-inflammatories, bicarbonate, and caffeine is recommended. Dehydration can also precipitate runner's diarrhea. Further study regarding dietary recommendations is ongoing. Continued hydration and symptomatic care are the mainstays of treatment.[21]

A rare but serious GI complication of ultramarathon running is exercise-induced ischemic colitis. This typically presents with sharp, severe abdominal pain and loose stools. The stools are often melanotic or frankly bloody differentiating this more serious state from runner's diarrhea. It is thought the colitis occurs due to catecholamine release shunting blood from splenic system to muscle, coupled with dehydration creating gut hypoperfusion. Bloody stools should prompt immediate evacuation and IV fluid resuscitation.[22]

COLD INJURY

Low temperatures can put runners at risk for cold weather injuries. These include frostbite, frostnip, and chilblains. Frostbite is caused by intracellular and extracellular ice crystal formation in body tissue. The presence of ice crystals damages the cells by changing the osmotic gradients. The presentation for frostbite is divided into 2 categories: superficial and deep. Superficial frostbite encompasses first-degree and second-degree damage, while third and fourth degree are referred to as deep frostbite. Superficial frostbite will have a pale or yellow patch of raised skin, often with decreased sensation. Deep frostbite involves the complete freezing of the skin along with deeper tissue layers. The affected area will develop blisters filled with hemorrhagic fluid.

Field treatment of frostbite requires prevention of further freezing. Rewarming should not be initiated if there is a chance of refreezing. To rewarm, the affected area is submerged in circulating water between 98°F and 102°F for 15 to 30 minutes. Monitor the area for return of pliability of the skin. If warm circulating water is not available, the area can be passively rewarmed by getting into a warmed structure or vehicle. Do not rewarm over open fire, as the tissue is at risk to burns due to decreased sensation. Rewarming may be painful and analgesia should be considered.

Frostnip is similar to frostbite, but the affected area will still be pliable on examination. Frostnip is a precursor to frostbite. It generally affects the fingers, toes, ears, and nose and occurs from exposure to cold temperatures without the tissue freezing. Rewarm the area as soon as possible.

Chilblains occurs at temperatures between 32°F and 59°F. Runners are more susceptible to developing chilblains when they have beenexposed to water. The runners will present with itchy, painful bumps, most often on the lower extremities, fingers, nose, and back. The symptoms can be improved with getting the affected area warm and dry, then covering it with a dry bandage. Benadryl is helpful for the itching.[23]

CORNEAL EDEMA

Ultramarathon-induced corneal edema (UMICE) is a transient, painless vision loss. Its starts with blurry vision and can progress to full blindness. It worsens during exercise, however, spontaneously resolves in hours to days. Although not well understood, the pathophysiology is proposed to be a lactate build up in the cornea due to corneal irritation and systemic rise in lactic acid. Racers with history of refractive surgery have a higher risk. Use of lubricating drops and protective eyewear seems to decrease the incidence.[24]

COMMUNICATION TECHNIQUES

Organized endurance events fall into the category of mass gatherings. The World Health Organization (WHO) defines mass gatherings as *"an organized or unplanned event where the number of people attending is sufficient to strain the planning and response resources of the community, state, or nation, hosting the event."* Events with more than 1000 participants are required to follow the National Incident Management structure developed by Homeland Security.[25] Free online training and certification for Incident Management are available on the Homeland Security website (https://www.firstrespondertraining.gov/frts/npcc).

In both large and small events, the use of the Incident Command Structure utilizing a preplanned, top down, communication structure, with 1 incident commander can be useful. The incident commander is responsible for devising pre-planned action plans/protocols for events likely to occur during the specific event, and communicating with local EMS. The race director and medical director work closely to develop medical protocols, communication strategies, and emergency response procedures to ensure safe and timely response to emergencies.[26]

Seamless communication on race day is essential for personnel to stay organized and respond efficiently to any emergency that may occur. Cellular towers can be overloaded during increased utilization causing communication to break down. In more austere environments, cellular coverage may be inconsistent. Utilization of radios allows open communication between race personnel, yet some limitations do exist. Radio waves travel primarily by *"line of sight,"* and thus may be impeded by mountains, ridges, or large structures. For this reason, radio repeaters may be utilized or placed in critical areas to facilitate radio communication around obstacles. Utilization of a preplanned communication structure, designating 1 radio operator as Network Control through which all radio traffic passes, allows for orderly communication. Many cities have local amateur radio clubs whose members are very knowledgeable and helpful in radio communication techniques.

SUMMARY

Providing medical support for ultra endurance running events is an exciting and satisfying way to contribute to a community. It is important to be organized and thorough in pre-race planning in order to ensure timely and effective care to the injured runner. The medical kit should be supplied/designed to care for diseases likely to be encountered for the specific race setting. In order to build an adequate medical kit, it is useful to categorize disease processes into *"serious but uncommon,"* and *"less serious but common,"'* and then outline specific supplies needed for each disease process. Finally, a preplanned communication structure and robust race day communication strategy is imperative to maintain an organized structure and effective response to race medical emergencies.

DISCLOSURE

The authors have nothing to disclose.

REFERENCES

1. Larson HH, Khalili-Borna D, Uzosike E, et al. Medical coverage of ultramarathons and its unique challenges. Curr Sports Med Rep 2016;15(3). https://doi.org/10.1249/JSR.0000000000000267.
2. Hoffman MD. Participant Opinions and Expectations about Medical Services at Ultramarathons: Findings from the Ultrarunners Longitudinal TRAcking (ULTRA) Study. Cureus 2019. https://doi.org/10.7759/cureus.5800.
3. Dallam GM, Jonas S, Miller TK. Medical considerations in triathlon competition: Recommendations for triathlon organisers, competitors and coaches. Sports Med 2005;35(2). https://doi.org/10.2165/00007256-200535020-00004.
4. Martinez MW, Kim JH, Shah AB, et al. Exercise-Induced Cardiovascular Adaptations and Approach to Exercise and Cardiovascular Disease: JACC State-of-the-Art Review. J Am Coll Cardiol 2021;78(14). https://doi.org/10.1016/j.jacc.2021.08.003.
5. Kinoshi T, Tanaka S, Sagisaka R, et al. Mobile Automated External Defibrillator Response System during Road Races. N Engl J Med 2018;379(5). https://doi.org/10.1056/nejmc1803218.
6. Gerow M, Bruner PJ. Exercise Induced Asthma. In: StatPearls [Internet]. Treasure Island (FL): StatPearls Publishing; 2023.
7. Atchley TJ, Smith DM. Exercise-induced bronchoconstriction in elite or endurance athletes:: Pathogenesis and diagnostic considerations. Ann Allergy Asthma Immunol 2020;125(1). https://doi.org/10.1016/j.anai.2020.01.023.
8. Gaudio FG, Johnson DE, DiLorenzo K, et al. Wilderness Medical Society Clinical Practice Guidelines on Anaphylaxis. Wilderness Environ Med 2022;33(1). https://doi.org/10.1016/j.wem.2021.11.009.
9. Hawkins SC, Weil C, Baty F, et al. Retrieval of additional epinephrine from auto-injectors. Wilderness Environ Med 2013;24(4). https://doi.org/10.1016/j.wem.2013.03.025.
10. Murray B, Rosenbloom C. Fundamentals of glycogen metabolism for coaches and athletes. Nutr Rev 2018;76(4). https://doi.org/10.1093/NUTRIT/NUY001.
11. Klingert M, Nikolaidis PT, Weiss K, et al. Exercise-associated hyponatremia in marathon runners. J Clin Med 2022;11(22):6775. https://doi.org/10.3390/jcm11226775.
12. Hew-Butler T, Loi V, Pani A, et al. Exercise-associated hyponatremia: 2017 update. Front Med 2017;4(MAR). https://doi.org/10.3389/fmed.2017.00021.

13. Giesbrecht GG. "Cold card" to guide responders in the assessment and care of cold-exposed patients. Wilderness Environ Med 2018;29(4). https://doi.org/10.1016/j.wem.2018.07.001.

14. Gomes YE, Chau M, Banwell HA, et al. Diagnostic accuracy of the Ottawa ankle rule to exclude fractures in acute ankle injuries in adults: a systematic review and meta-analysis. BMC Muscoskel Disord 2022;23(1):885. https://doi.org/10.1186/s12891-022-05831-7.

15. Krabak BJ, Waite B, Schiff MA. Study of injury and illness rates in multiday ultra-marathon runners. Med Sci Sports Exerc 2011;43(12). https://doi.org/10.1249/MSS.0b013e318221bfe3.

16. Lipman GS, Ellis MA, Lewis EJ, et al. A Prospective Randomized Blister Prevention Trial Assessing Paper Tape in Endurance Distances (Pre-TAPED). Wilderness Environ Med 2014;25(4). https://doi.org/10.1016/j.wem.2014.06.013.

17. Cortese TA, Fukuyama K, Epstein W, et al. Treatment of Friction Blisters: An Experimental Study. Arch Dermatol 1968;97(6). https://doi.org/10.1001/archderm.1968.01610120107016.

18. Brennan FH. Managing blisters in competitive athletes. Curr Sports Med Rep 2002;1(6). https://doi.org/10.1249/00149619-200212000-00003.

19. Huang YH, Hsieh TY, Chen IC, et al. Amputation of lower limb for necrotizing soft-tissue infection in an ultramarathon runner. Formosan Journal of Surgery 2014;47(2). https://doi.org/10.1016/j.fjs.2013.10.003.

20. van Wijck K, Lenaerts K, Grootjans J, et al. Physiology and pathophysiology of splanchnic hypoperfusion and intestinal injury during exercise: Strategies for evaluation and prevention. Am J Physiol Gastrointest Liver Physiol 2012;303(2). https://doi.org/10.1152/ajpgi.00066.2012.

21. de Oliveira EP. Runner's diarrhea. Curr Opin Gastroenterol 2017;33(1):41–6. https://doi.org/10.1097/MOG.0000000000000322.

22. Faress A, Masood S, Mian A. "Runs" from a run: A case of exercise induced ischemic colitis. World J Emerg Med 2017;8(4). https://doi.org/10.5847/wjem.j.1920-8642.2017.04.010.

23. Ingram BJ, Raymond TJ. Recognition and treatment of freezing and nonfreezing cold injuries. Curr Sports Med Rep 2013;12(2). https://doi.org/10.1249/JSR.0b013e3182877454.

24. Lindström BE, Høeg TB. Ultramarathon-induced Corneal Edema - A Case Report. Curr Sports Med Rep 2021;20(1). https://doi.org/10.1249/JSR.0000000000000796.

25. McCarthy DM, Chiampas GT, Malik S, et al. Enhancing community disaster resilience through mass sporting events. Disaster Med Public Health Prep 2011;5(4). https://doi.org/10.1001/dmp.2011.46.

26. Chiampas GT, Goyal AV. Innovative Operations Measures and Nutritional Support for Mass Endurance Events. Sports Med 2015;45. https://doi.org/10.1007/s40279-015-0396-6.

Medicine Above the Horizon
Altitude Medicine

Jessica Gehner, MD*

KEYWORDS

• Altitude related illness • HACE • HAPE

KEY POINTS

- Proper acclimatization is crucial in avoiding altitude-related illness. Acclimatization is optimized by a slow, gradual ascent profile and prophylaxis with medications such as acetazolamide.
- Diagnosis of altitude-related illness occurs most commonly in resource-limited environments. Acute mountain sickness is diagnosed based on history, whereas more severe manifestations of altitude illness such as high-altitude cerebral edema and high-altitude pulmonary edema have abnormal physical examination findings.
- The definitive treatment of all altitude-related illnesses is descent. Supplemental oxygen and pharmacologic treatment are temporizing measures until the patient can be evacuated to a lower altitude.

INTRODUCTION

So, if you cannot understand that there is something in man which responds to the challenge of this mountain and goes out to meet it, that the struggle is the struggle of life itself upward and forever upward, then you won't see why we go. What we get from this adventure is just sheer joy. And joy is, after all, the end of life.
—*George Mallory*

Climbers, mountaineers, and trekkers are often asked why they intentionally place themselves in such a dangerous and harsh environment just to stand on a summit. "Because it's there" is the resounding answer. Yet, even the most experienced and well-trained athletes are not immune to the effects of high altitude. The author reviews the physiologic response to high altitude as well as the spectrum of altitude-related illness, how to treat it and when it is necessary to descend.

HISTORY/DEFINITIONS/BACKGROUND

One does not have to be summiting Everest to be at risk for altitude-related illness. Elevations above 1500 m (4,921 ft) are considered high altitude. Above 3500 m

---

Department of Emergency Medicine, Roanoke, VA, USA
* 4759 Mountain View Church Road, Blue Ridge, VA 24064.
E-mail address: jrgehner@carilionclinic.org

Physician Assist Clin 9 (2024) 291–302
https://doi.org/10.1016/j.cpha.2023.09.001
2405-7991/24/© 2023 Elsevier Inc. All rights reserved.

(11,483 ft) is considered very high altitude, and elevations greater than 5500 m (18,045 ft) are considered extreme altitude. While still possible, it is extremely rare to see altitude-related illness below 2500 m (8,200 ft).[1]

As altitude increases, the barometric pressure decreases, also decreasing the partial pressure of inhaled oxygen. The result is a hypobaric hypoxia, which is the driving force for the physiologic changes seen with acclimatization, the process of our bodies becoming accustomed to this low-oxygen environment. When the body does not properly acclimatize, conditions such as acute mountain sickness (AMS), high-altitude cerebral edema (HACE) and high-altitude pulmonary edema (HAPE) may occur. AMS and HACE can be thought of as a spectrum of disease with HACE being the most severe manifestation.

ACCLIMATIZATION

Acclimatization occurs in two phases: acute and chronic. Within hours of arrival to high altitude, the hypoxic ventilatory response increases the respiratory rate leading to a respiratory alkalosis. This improves oxygenation by decreasing the partial pressure of carbon dioxide in the alveoli but also causes an alkalosis. The kidneys respond to this increased pH by secreting bicarbonate in the urine causing a diuresis. This diuresis causes hemoconcentration, thereby increasing hematocrit. The increase in hematocrit is due to decreased water content in the blood during the acute phase of acclimatization. Adequate diuresis is associated with proper acclimatization. Acetazolamide facilitates this process by secreting bicarbonate ions into the urine and decreasing the blood pH. The pH-sensitive respiratory centers in the brain then respond to the more acidic environment with an increased respiratory rate.

After 3 to 4 weeks at high altitude, increased erythropoietin production results in increased red blood cell (RBC) mass from the manufacture of new RBCs further increasing the hematocrit. Full acclimatization usually takes 4 to 6 weeks but varies greatly based on multiple factors: rate of ascent, geographic location, and physiologic differences in populations.[2] This is the rationale behind climbers living at a high-altitude base camp for weeks before attempting high summits such as Mt Everest.

PATHOPHYSIOLOGY

When proper acclimatization does not occur, patients may develop altitude-related illness, AMS, HACE, or HAPE. Each of these disease processes is ultimately a result of hypobaric hypoxia, relative hypoventilation, increased sympathetic drive, and fluid redistribution. The pathophysiology of AMS is not totally understood, and several hypotheses are still being studied to further delineate this very subjective and nebulous disease process. Some experts discuss the *"leaky-vessel theory"* in which inflammation from hypoxia increases endothelin and causes fluid to leak from blood vessels into the interstitium. In a more severe form, the edema can result in HACE or HAPE. This is one reason that nonsteroid anti-inflammatory drugs (NSAIDs) have been explored as a possible preventative and/or treatment option.[1]

Relative hypoventilation contributes to the symptoms of altitude illness as well as the sleep apnea that many people experience when visiting high altitudes. Chemoreceptors in the respiratory centers of the brain are pH-sensitive. This decreases the respiratory rate in response to a high pH and increases respiratory rate when the pH is low. If acclimatization is inadequate or alkalosis too extreme, respiratory rate can decrease even to the point of apnea while asleep, causing not only lower peripheral oxygen saturation (SpO_2) but also very poor sleep at high altitude.

EPIDEMIOLOGY

The incidence and severity of AMS depend on the rate of ascent and altitude attained (especially sleeping altitude), duration of altitude exposure, level of exertion, recent altitude exposure, and genetic susceptibility.[3] One of the most predictive factors is a previous history of AMS. The incidence of AMS ranges from 5% to 68% depending on the rate of ascent or gain in altitude. The incidence of HACE is approximately 1% and the incidence of HAPE is approximately 2%.[4]

Altitude of residence also plays a role in the incidence of AMS. Those living at ≥900m had an 8% incidence of AMS compared with 27% incidence those living at sea level.[5] Age may be a protective factor for AMS; one study shows age greater than 60 years had half the incidence when compared with younger patients.[6] One hypothesis for this finding is that cerebral atrophy provides additional room in the skull to accommodate swelling. Children and young adults seem to be equally susceptible to AMS, whereas women may have the same or a slightly higher incidence of AMS.[6,7] Obesity seems to increase the risk of developing AMS.[5] However, physical fitness is not a predictor of susceptibility to AMS. Elite athletes are often willing to push through extreme discomfort and ultimately may become much more ill before alerting others to their distress (**Fig. 1**).

PREVENTION OF ALTITUDE-RELATED ILLNESS

Travel to high-altitude locations often involves extensive training, planning, expensive gear, and precious time (**Fig. 2**). Countless trekkers and mountaineers have had to abort their trips due to altitude-related illness. Others have proceeded despite concerning symptoms and dangerous conditions and lost their lives. Although many of us may never work in a clinical setting where we are treating altitude-related complaints, one thing we can do is counsel patients on how to prevent altitude-related illness in the first place.

GRADED ASCENT

"Climb high, sleep low;" sleeping elevation is the most important consideration when planning a high-altitude expedition. In order to prevent AMS, the Wilderness Medical Society (WMS) Clinical Practice Guidelines recommend that one does not increase their sleeping elevation by ≤ 500 m/day. An acclimatization day (in which there is NO gain in sleeping elevation) should be taken for every 1000 m gained. If routes and logistics require that more than 500 m elevation is gained in a day, an extra acclimatization day should be taken to simulate a more gradual ascent.[8] Although rest and refueling are important, taking a short hike on those days is a common practice and may aid in acclimatization.

PHARMACOLOGIC PROPHYLAXIS

In those with a higher likelihood of suffering from AMS (ie, steep ascent profile, those with a history of AMS), prophylaxis should be considered. The first line medication in both the treatment and prevention of AMS is acetazolamide. Prophylaxis should start 24 hours before ascent. A dose of 125 mg twice/day orally is the current

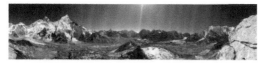

Fig. 1. Everest Panorama. (Photo courtesy of Jessie Gehner, used with permission.)

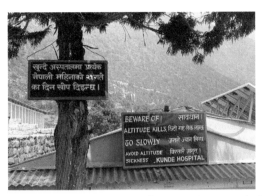

Fig. 2. Kunde Hospital, Nepal. (Photo courtesy of Jessie Gehner, used with permission.)

recommendation, though lower doses have recently shown to be effective. More data are needed to validate these results.[9]

In those who cannot take acetazolamide, dexamethasone (2 mg orally every 6 hours) can also be used as prophylaxis. Using steroids as prophylaxis can result in adrenal insufficiency if taken for more than 10 days and not tapered. It is also theorized that the treatment of HACE with dexamethasone may be less effective if one is already taking corticosteroids.

Several studies have looked at using NSAIDs such as ibuprofen for prevention of AMS. Trekkers taking 600 mg of ibuprofen three times daily had overall higher oxygen saturations than the control group.[10] Ibuprofen can be used for AMS prevention in persons who do not wish to take acetazolamide or dexamethasone or have allergies or intolerance to these medications.[8]

Numerous natural remedies, including ginger tea, ginkgo biloba, and coca leaves, have been recommended for centuries by locals living at high altitude to prevent altitude sickness and improve acclimatization. Studies are extremely limited on these substances and there are no formal recommendations for their use.

For patients with a history of HAPE, or for those who may be at higher risk, prophylactic nifedipine can be given (30 mg extended-release orally every 12 hours). Other medications, such as sildenafil, tadalafil, and salmeterol which are used in treatment, have been evaluated for prophylaxis, but their use is not recommended.[8]

ADEQUATE HYDRATION

A person exerting themselves at high altitude has many reasons to be dehydrated. Fluid losses due to increased respiration, sweating, and/or diuretic use (if on acetazolamide) all contribute to dehydration. This is often compounded by poor oral intake due to a low thirst drive in the cold and/or nausea. Many trekking guides encourage their clients to drink copious amounts of water at high altitude, which can result in fluid overload and hyponatremia. The WMS consensus guidelines recommend drinking to thirst and watching urine coloration.[8] Addition of electrolyte mix can also be helpful when overall oral intake is poor.

DIAGNOSIS

The diagnosis of the below disease processes will often be made in an austere, resource-limited environment (as with most wilderness medicine-related conditions). For this reason, a thorough history and physical examination may be your only guide. Although it is important to keep a broad differential diagnosis, it should be assumed that signs and symptoms are altitude-related until proven otherwise and descent should be planned.

ACUTE MOUNTAIN SICKNESS

The diagnosis of AMS is subjective and not based on any specific findings on physical examination, laboratory work, or imaging. The first symptom required to be present is headache, which is often accompanied by other symptoms, nausea, anorexia, fatigue, dizziness, and/or difficulty sleeping. Symptom onset occurs 6 to 12 hours after arrival at high altitude.

The Lake Louise AMS Score is the sum of the severity ratings of the below symptoms (**Fig. 3**). AMS score should be calculated only after 6 hours after arrival to high altitude, to avoid confusing AMS with confounding symptoms from travel or responses to acute hypoxia. Other conditions on the differential diagnosis include dehydration, migraine headache, hyponatremia, or viral illness.

Treatment of Acute Mountain Sickness

The definitive treatment for all altitude-related disorders is descent. The treatments discussed below are only temporizing measures until a safe descent can be made. Remote locations, communication difficulties, dangerous weather, and rough terrain may make a timely evacuation impossible. Most symptoms typically improve or resolve after a descent of 300 to 1000 m, but the required decrease in altitude varies among individuals.[8]

The symptoms of mild to moderate AMS may be treated in the backcountry without mandating descent; however, a patient with AMS should not continue to ascend until symptoms improve. One strategy is taking an extra acclimatization day while starting the treatment dose of acetazolamide (250 mg twice a day), giving medications to treat the symptoms of AMS (NSAIDs, antiemetics) and ensuring adequate hydration. Supplemental oxygen can be used if available. If the patient's symptoms improve, they may consider continuing their trip at high altitude while continuing the treatment dose of acetazolamide.

Severe AMS mandates descent. Supplemental oxygen should be initiated, and acetazolamide and other symptom controlling medications should be administered. Owing to the nausea and vomiting that often are present in severe AMS, parenteral antiemetics

Acute Mountain Sickness

Symptom	Headache	GI symptoms	Fatigue Weakness	Dizziness Lightheadedness	Function
	None = 0	None = 0	Not tired = 0	No dizziness = 0	No change in plans
	Mild = 1	Poor appetite Nausea = 1	Mild fatigue = 1	Mild dizziness = 1	Symptoms present, no change in plans
	Mod = 2	Mod nausea Vomiting = 2	Mod fatigue, weakness = 2	Mod dizziness = 2	Symptoms forced descent under own power
	Severe = 3	Severe nausea, vomiting = 3	Severe fatigue incapacitating = 3	Severe dizziness Incapacitating = 3	Had to be evacuated to lower altitude

Fig. 3. Acute Mountain Sickness (AMS) present if headache score of >1 point, with mild defined as 3-5 points, Moderate defined as 6-9 points and severe AMS defined as 10-12 points. Based on the Lake Louise Mountain Sickness Score* (*Adapted from* International Society of Mountain Medicine, Roach RC, et al for the Lake Louise AMS Score Consensus Committee. The 2018 Lake Louise Acute Mountain Sickness Score. High Alt Med Biol. 2018 Mar;19(1):4-6.)

can be useful (ie, ondansetron oral dissolving tablet [ODT], promethazine rectal suppositories).[8] The patient should be monitored closely for any neurologic signs and not be allowed to descend independently in case they progress from severe AMS to HACE. On prolonged treks or travel to very high altitude, AMS can still occur on descent. Acetazolamide may be initiated at the treatment dose even while descending.

HIGH-ALTITUDE CEREBRAL EDEMA

HACE is diagnosed in a patient presenting with the symptoms of severe AMS with a neurologic deficit, ataxia, visual changes, altered mental status, seizures, or in cases of impending cerebral herniation, a comatose state. The classic patient with HACE may seem to be intoxicated, slurring their speech, unable to walk in a straight line, vomiting, with altered mental status.

The use of portable ultrasound is becoming more common in austere environments, and ocular ultrasound may reveal increased diameter of the optic nerve sheath.[11] Nerve sheath diameters of less than 0.55 cm are indicative of increased intracranial pressure (**Fig. 4**). In the rare cases where MRI was used on patients with HACE, the findings were consistent with vasogenic edema. Other conditions that should be on the differential include intracranial hemorrhage, ischemic stroke, seizure disorder, atypical migraine, intoxication, and other metabolic disturbances.

TREATMENT OF HIGH-ALTITUDE CEREBRAL EDEMA

Supplemental oxygen is a mainstay of treatment for AMS, HACE, and HAPE. When supplemental oxygen is unavailable, a Gamow bag (portable hyperbaric chamber)

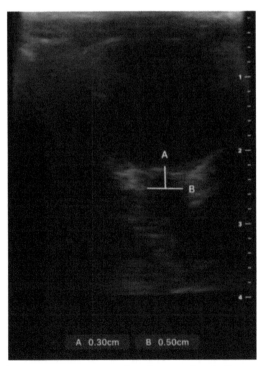

Fig. 4. Ultrasound showing measurements of optic nerve sheath diameter. (Ultrasound used with permission of Jessie Gehner.)

can simulate a decrease in altitude by thousands of feet while awaiting evacuation and descent. Gamow bags are fraught with difficulties, however, including the need for constant pumping of a foot pedal by an attendant and the inability to closely monitor a critical patient.[12]

HACE can rapidly progress to herniation and death, so immediate descent is indicated for any neurologic abnormality at high altitude. Supplemental oxygen should be administered and if unavailable, the patient should be placed in a Gamow bag while waiting for descent. Dexamethasone should be administered (8 mg initial dose followed by 4 mg every 6 hour can be given orally, subcutaneously or intravenously). Acetazolamide should also be considered, given at the treatment dose (250 mg twice a day).[8] Treating symptomatic patients with NSAIDs and antiemetics should also be considered. HACE patients may be altered and uncooperative making treatment extremely difficult. As with severe AMS, these patients should be monitored closely and not left alone.

HIGH-ALTITUDE PULMONARY EDEMA

The diagnosis of HAPE can be made if the patient has at least two of the following symptoms: chest tightness or pain, cough, and dyspnea at rest or decreased exercise tolerance. In addition, two or more of the following examination findings must be present: central cyanosis, rales/wheezes, tachycardia, or tachypnea.[13] Time of onset for HAPE usually occurs 2 to 4 days after arrival at high altitude.

If available, chest xray may show patchy alveolar infiltrates with normal-sized mediastinum/heart. An ultrasound may show B-lines consistent with pulmonary edema (**Fig. 5**). ECG may show signs of right axis deviation and/or ischemia. Labs are of limited utility. HAPE patients are very quickly responsive to supplemental oxygen.

The classic HAPE patient will be extremely dyspneic, complain of orthopnea with crackles on auscultation and may have a cough productive of pink, frothy sputum. Other conditions that should be on the differential diagnosis include pulmonary embolism, cardiomyopathy, pneumonia, or congestive heart failure.

TREATMENT OF HIGH-ALTITUDE PULMONARY EDEMA

As with other altitude-related disorders, the best treatment for HAPE is rapid descent. Supplemental oxygen and Gamow bags can be used while awaiting evacuation. HAPE can be similar in appearance to pulmonary edema precipitated by heart failure, but the treatments are not identical. Diuretics such as furosemide are not recommended.

The goals of treatment of HAPE are to improve oxygenation and reduce resistance in the pulmonary vasculature. First-line therapy is nifedipine (30 mg sustained release twice a day). Other therapies to reduce pulmonary vascular resistance include phosphodiesterase inhibitors such as tadalafil or sildenafil. While sometimes used in treatment, inhaled beta agonists have not been shown to be effective, but are not likely harmful.[8]

CONCURRENT HIGH-ALTITUDE CEREBRAL EDEMA AND HIGH-ALTITUDE PULMONARY EDEMA

Again, rapid descent is mandatory. Supplemental oxygen or Gamow bag should be used until descent can be made. Dexamethasone should be added to the above treatment regimen for HAPE. It may be difficult to discern whether neurologic dysfunction is due to hypoxic encephalopathy or from HACE in the backcountry, so it is important to treat both entities if the patient meets criteria. Although phosphodiesterase inhibitors

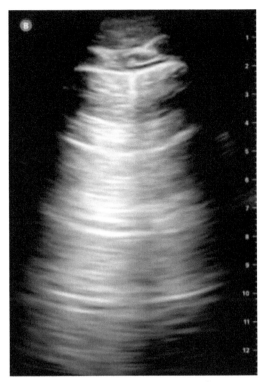

Fig. 5. Ultrasound showing B-lines consistent with pulmonary edema. (Ultrasound used with permission of Jessie Gehner.)

and calcium channel blockers are not contraindicated in HACE treatment, patients should be monitored closely for hypotension. A decrease in cerebral perfusion pressure may worsen ischemia if it is present.

Other Altitude-Related Conditions

Retinal/vitreous hemorrhage
Hypoxia at high altitude brings about retinal neovascular changes. Increased blood pressure during strenuous work at altitude can increase the pressure in retinal blood vessels, resulting in capillary leaks and subsequent high-altitude retinal hemorrhage.[14] These findings can be seen on ophthalmoscopy and sometimes on ultrasound. Patients should be counseled to avoid exertion if vision changes are present and should have close ophthalmologic follow-up.

High-altitude cough
Sometimes called the *"Khumbu cough,"* this nonproductive, persistent, paroxysmal cough is common and quite bothersome to many high-altitude travelers. The cough can be so severe that it causes rib fractures. Although the exact etiology is not clearly understood, the commonly held belief that it was due solely to the inspiration of cold, dry air was refuted by observations and experiments in long duration hypobaric chamber studies. High-altitude cough is likely a symptom of several possible perturbations in the cough reflex arc that may exist independently or together. These include loss of

water from the respiratory tract, respiratory tract infections, or subclinical HAPE.[15] Silica in dust has also been implicated as a cause of the *Khumbu cough* as many trekkers inhale this sparkling dust while on their journey. Wearing a moist facial covering so that particulate matter is filtered and inspired air is warmed/moistened may prevent or decrease this troublesome symptom.

Chronic mountain sickness

This illness is seen in patients with long-term residence at altitude greater than 3000 m (10,000 ft) above sea level. It is insidious in onset, presenting with increasing weakness, shortness of breath (SOB), fatigue, somnolence, and slowed mental functioning. It can progress to complete incapacitation. Chronic mountain sickness (CMS) is characterized by severe symptomatic erythrocytosis (Hemoglobin [Hgb] $\geq$19 g/dL for women and Hgb $\geq$21 g/dL for men) and accentuated hypoxemia, frequently associated with pulmonary hypertension. In advanced cases, the condition may evolve to cor pulmonale and congestive heart failure.[16] Patients with suspected CMS should be evaluated at a facility, where cardiology and pulmonology can diagnose and manage sequelae (heart failure, pulmonary hypertension, or thrombosis).

CASE STUDY: A 34-YEAR-OLD WOMAN WITH HEADACHE

- *History of Present Illness*: A 34-year-old woman presents with headache, anorexia, vomiting, light headedness, and fatigue. She is on day 9 of a trek to Everest Base Camp (EBC) at 5125 m (16,814 ft). The ascent profile has been gradual taking acclimatization days at 3840 m (12,598 ft) and 4410 m (14,470 ft). She complains of a worsening headache for the past 24 hours, anorexia, fatigue, and dizziness. She denies any weakness or numbness, but does have paresthesias in her hands and feet. She reports some visual disturbance (floaters/blurriness) but denies vomiting, diarrhea, and chest pain. She reports mild SOB, which has been present since arrival at high altitude. When it is suggested to this patent that she may have AMS, she insists that this is a migraine headache.
- *Past Medical History*: Migraine headaches, anorexia nervosa, is an endurance athlete. Maximum altitude reached on previous treks 15,000 ft without significant symptoms.
- *Medications*: 125 mg acetazolamide twice a day orally for prophylaxis initiated 24 hours before the start of her trek
- *Allergies*: none

PHYSICAL EXAMINATION

Vital Signs: Heart rate 125 beats/min, SPO_2 85%, respiratory rate 25, BP (not available), temp (not available)

General: Alert, oriented, appears fatigued.

HEENT: Mucous membranes dry, no other abnormalities.

Cardiac: Radial pulse 2+ bilaterally, regular.

Respiratory: Mild tachypnea, no audible wheezing or crackles.

Skin: Pale, cool, dry, no cyanosis.

Neuro: No focal deficits.

Patient was started on treatment dose of acetazolamide (250 mg twice/day), ondansetron (4 mg ODT), and ibuprofen (600 mg three times/day). She was encouraged to increase her oral fluid intake, although patient was reluctant due to feeling unwell. Her team is scheduled to leave for EBC in the morning.

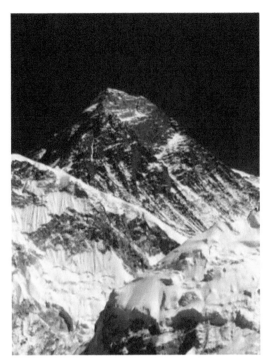

Fig. 6. Mt Everest, Tibet Autonomous Region, Khumbu Valley, Nepal. (Photo used with permission of Jessie Gehner.)

In the morning, the patient's symptoms had worsened, although she is still without focal neurologic symptoms. Despite medication, her headache has worsened. It is recommended that the patient descend and not proceed to EBC. She says that this is her regular migraine headache and she is not turning back.

One hour into the trek, the patient becomes more fatigued and ataxic. She begins slurring her speech. The headache continues to worsen. She is given dexamethasone 8 mg orally but immediately vomits. Fortunately, another team has injectable dexamethasone and she is subsequently given 8 mg intramuscularly.

Patient could ambulate and so with the help of her team mates, she is walked down to 4940 m (16,000 ft) where she is evacuated by helicopter to Kathmandu. By the time she arrives, at the receiving facility, her symptoms have almost completely resolved.

DISCUSSION

Because this patient had a history of migraine headaches, she was reluctant to descend, blaming her symptoms on her migraines rather than AMS. This was complicated by her desire to reach her destination for which she had extensively trained, planned, and spent a great deal of money.

The patient started out with moderate AMS. She was treated appropriately, however, because she did not descend, it progressed to severe AMS by the next morning. Once neurologic signs became present (ataxia, slurred speech) patient met the criteria for HACE.

She could not tolerate PO dexamethasone due to her nausea and vomiting, and so it was potentially lifesaving that she could receive it intramuscularly. Her teammates also took advantage of her ability to continue to ambulate on her own and assisted her to a lower altitude immediately. It would have been a much more prolonged extrication should she have had to be carried, delaying her descent to a lower altitude potentially resulting in a different outcome. Air evacuation was available, but this is not always an option when visibility is limited.

Although it is important to keep a broad differential diagnosis, one could not safely say that it was a complex migraine at high altitude. The quick resolution of her symptoms on arrival to Kathmandu at 1340 m (4,396 ft) suggests that the patient had HACE.

SUMMARY

Travel to high altitude can be one of the most beautiful, breathtaking experiences of one's life (**Fig. 6**). It also can be the most dangerous. Diagnostics and treatment options are extremely limited in most cases and altitude-related illness should be assumed until proven otherwise. Care should be taken when counseling patients before high-altitude travel so that they are educated about high-altitude illness, which medications should be taken and when, and most importantly, when to descend. In travelers who have planned a rapid ascent or have a history of altitude-related illness, pharmacologic prophylaxis should be considered. Most of all, the mountains should be respected, not only for their grandeur but also for their awesome power to destroy. The prudent mountain enthusiast must know when to push on and when to turn back.

Getting to the top is optional. Getting down is mandatory.

CLINICS CARE POINTS

- If altitude illness is suspected, the definitive treatment is DESCENT.
- Pharmacologic agents and supplemental oxygen are only temporizing measures until descent is accomplished.
- Concerning symptoms should be considered altitude-related until proven otherwise and diagnostics should not delay descent.
- Patients with even mild symptoms of acute mountain sickness (AMS) should not continue to ascend until symptoms have improved.
- Oxygen saturation does not always correlate with the severity of disease; consider the entire clinical picture including the patient's functional status.
- Graded ascent limited to 500 m/24-h period and a lower altitude sleeping elevation each night is recommended to prevent altitude-related illness.
- Acetazolamide is the first-line medication for both treatment and prevention of AMS.
- Small, portable ultrasound is becoming more common as a diagnostic tool in the backcountry and can help the practitioner diagnose conditions including high-altitude cerebral edema and high-altitude pulmonary edema.
- While it is important to keep a broad differential diagnosis when evaluating the patient with suspected altitude-related illness, symptoms must be attributed to the high-altitude environment until proven otherwise. Descent should be anticipated and arranged.

DISCLOSURES

The author has nothing to disclose.

REFERENCES

1. Auerbach PS, Cushing TA, Stuart Harris N. Auerbach's wilderness medicine. Elsevier; 2017.
2. Waeber B, Kayser B, Dumont L, et al. Impact of study design on reported incidences of acute mountain sickness: a systematic review. High Alt Med Biol 2015;16(3):204–15.
3. Bloch KE, Latshang TD, Turk AJ, et al. Nocturnal periodic breathing during acclimatization at very high altitude at Mount Muztagh Ata (7,546 m). Am J Respir Crit Care Med 2010;182(4):562–8.
4. Basnyat B, Subedi D, Sleggs J, et al. Disoriented and ataxic pilgrims: an epidemiological study of acute mountain sickness and high-altitude cerebral edema at a sacred lake at 4300 m in the Nepal Himalayas. Wilderness Environ Med 2000; 11(2):89–93.
5. Honigman B, Theis MK, Koziol-McLain J, et al. Acute mountain sickness in a general tourist population at moderate altitudes. Ann Intern Med 1993;118:587–92.
6. Schneider M, Bernasch D, Weymann J, et al. Acute mountain sickness: Influence of susceptibility, preexposure, and ascent rate. Med Sci Sports Exerc 2002;34:1886–91.
7. Wu T. Children on the Tibetan plateau. ISSM Newslett 1994;4:5–7.
8. Luks AM, Auerbach PS, Freer L, et al. Wilderness medical society practice guidelines for the prevention and treatment of acute altitude illness: 2019 Update. Wilderness Environ Med 2019;30(4). https://doi.org/10.1016/j.wem.2019.04.006.
9. McIntosh SE, Hemphill M, McDevitt MC, et al. Reduced acetazolamide dosing in countering altitude illness: a comparison of 62.5 vs 125 mg (the RADICAL Trial). Wilderness Environ Med 2019;30(1):12–21.
10. Kanaan NC, Peterson AL, Pun M, et al. Prophylactic acetaminophen or ibuprofen result in equivalent acute mountain sickness incidence at high altitude: a prospective randomized trial. Wilderness Environ Med 2017;28(2):72–8.
11. Kanaan NC, Lipman GS, Constance BB, et al. Optic nerve sheath diameter increase on ascent to high altitude: correlation with acute mountain sickness. J Ultrasound Med 2015;34(9):1677–82.
12. Taber RL. Protocols for the use of a portable hyperbaric chamber for the treatment of high altitude disorders. J Wilderness Med 1990;1(3):181–92.
13. Jensen JD, Vincent AL. High altitude pulmonary edema. PubMed. Published 2021. Accessed December 2, 2021. https://www.ncbi.nlm.nih.gov/books/NBK430819/.
14. Wiedman M, Tabin GC. High-altitude retinopathy and altitude illness. Ophthalmology 1999;106(10):1924–7.
15. Mason NP. Altitude-related cough. Cough 2013;9(1):23.
16. Villafuerte FC, Corante N. Chronic mountain sickness: clinical aspects, etiology, management, and treatment. High Alt Med Biol 2016;17(2):61–9.

Medicine in the Heights
An Exploration of Mountain Medicine

Jason Pearce Beissinger, MS, PA-C, DiMM

KEYWORDS

- Mountain rescue • Wilderness EMS • Psychological first aid • Mountain medicine
- Climbing • Alpinism

KEY POINTS

- Mountain rescuers may come from all walks of life: carpentry, law, ministry, engineering, military, or even tailoring. Collectively, these teammates bring together their unique blend of skills that, along with medical and technical rescue training, prepare team member(s) to successfully execute a mountain rescue mission.
- The sacrifice of time for training and missions comes at the cost of personal pursuits.
- Practitioners are motivated by the greater good of volunteering for the sake of others.
- The uniqueness of physician assistants and nurse practitioners, along with their physician colleagues, brings together a resource to serve the rescue team and their mission in the mountains.

INTRODUCTION

In 1959, local rescuers gathered at Timberline Lodge on the flanks of Mt Hood, Oregon, to initiate a new culture in mountain rescue. This gathering led to the establishment of the Mountain Rescue Association (MRA). By upholding standards and accreditation for high-angle technical rescue teams, the MRA has made a tremendous use of medical providers to facilitate the advancement of its mission: *saving lives through rescue and mountain safety education*.[1,2] The uniqueness of physician assistant (PA) and nurse practitioner (NP) training, often as former rescue technicians, basic life support/advanced life support trainers, and providers of advanced medical care, has helped bridge the gap that often exists in rescue culture. By adding further training, Advanced Wilderness Life Support or the more substantial Diploma in Mountain Medicine (DiMM) further prepares these PAs and NPs for emergency care. Over recent years, the partnership of these providers working alongside their collaborating physician colleagues has led to the culture and development of Wilderness Emergency Medical Services.[3]

As such, PAs and NPs are often deployed into the field to allow advanced levels of medical care to be brought to the patient. This mitigates a potential delay of care

Portland Mountain Rescue, 13095 SE Snowfire Drive, Happy Valley, OR 97086, USA
E-mail address: beissinger@gmail.com

Physician Assist Clin 9 (2024) 303–310
https://doi.org/10.1016/j.cpha.2023.10.003
2405-7991/24/Published by Elsevier Inc.

physicianassistant.theclinics.com

required by patient packaging and extraction. Operating in the mountain rescue environment requires a situational awareness by all rescuers as the hazards in place may dictate different priorities than otherwise considered in front country medicine. Hasty removal from a hazard may indeed be the "best medicine" in caring for the patient.[4] Those rescuers trained in technical rigging and rope rescue will be challenged to balance the timing and delivery of care in concert with the mitigation of further patient injury.

Indeed, knowledge of the unique physiologic threats to patient viability must also be considered and is more aptly understood by medical providers.[2] This can include the generic considerations of orthopedic injuries and hypo/hyperthermia but may also include more complex considerations such as altitude physiology, metabolic chemistry, or even hazardous gas exposure.[5] High-altitude mountains and backcountry environments across the United States may present a need to recognize and care for patients suffering a variety of illnesses. The diversity of disease processes from high-altitude pulmonary edema (HAPE) and high-altitude cerebral edema (HACE) to envenomation and burns requires training. The Wilderness Medical Society (WMS) has developed guidelines for care (https://wms.org/magazine/1191/WMS_Clinical_Practice_Guidelines).[6]

For HAPE and HACE, these disease processes, even when mitigated by acclimatization, have specific management strategies. There are unique geological locations, that is, the Pacific Northwest cascade volcanoes that dictate further familiarization wilderness medicine. Within the cascade volcanic range, there is a risk of exposure to toxic gases and the resultant hazards presented to patients injured in volcanic fumaroles.[7] A fumarole is a vented opening in or near a volcano from which hazardous gasses such as hydrogen sulfide, carbon dioxide, or sulfur dioxide are emitted (**Fig. 1**).

The threat of these gasses requires a rescuer to attempt to decrease these hazards while successfully retrieving a patient who may have succumbed to their exposure— often with other simultaneous injuries. Such rescues demand special equipment such as air-purifying respirators (APRs), gas monitors, and technical rope systems rigged with additional contingencies (**Figs. 2 and 3**).[8]

Various agencies including the Occupational Safety and Health Administration set prescribed tolerances and limitations which must be taken into consideration by rescuers. Exposure breaching these established parameters may lead to apnea, asphyxiation, coma, dizziness, mucous membrane irritation, decreased visual acuity, nausea, and/or headaches.[9] Although generic appreciation of risk must be understood by all rescuers, a deeper understanding more complex elements is important for the medical rescuer. This includes the oxy-hemoglobin dissociation curve, pharmacokinetics, pharmacodynamics, and advanced patient assessment skills all of which aid providers in the

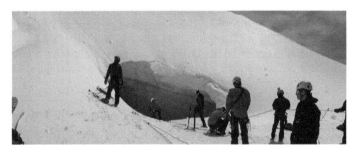

Fig. 1. Fumarole formed in Pacific Northwest Mountain Range. (*Courtesy of* Pearce Beissinger, used with permission; Fumarole, South Side of Mt Hood, Oregon.)

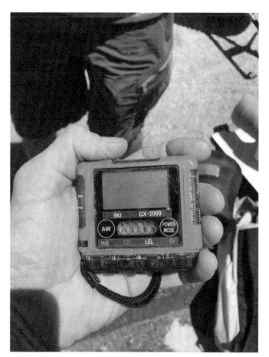

Fig. 2. Confined Space Gas Monitor(used in fumaroles) measures o2,H2S, CO, CO2 (oxygen, hydrogen sulfide, carbon monoxide, carbon dioxide) (*Courtesy of* Pearce Beissinger, used with permission; Fumarole, South Side of Mt Hood, Oregon.)

prioritization of field medical care and the resources that are being brought to the patient.

TRAINING

Training for the rigorous demands of mountain rescue may be accomplished by formal rope technician courses or internally within specific team-based curriculums. Patient

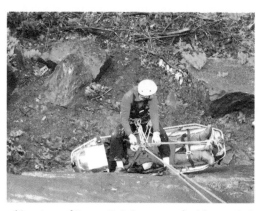

Fig. 3. Rrescue litter. (*Courtesy of* Pearce Beissinger, used with permission; Fumarole, South Side of Mt Hood, Oregon.)

packaging and litter positioning are two areas where advanced knowledge of medicine may dictate the processes by which technical rope rescue can be accomplished.[10] Understanding the mechanism of action for injury and patient assessment findings will often require variations of patient packaging. This can include a vacuum mattress versus a litter versus an SKED versus a screamer suit.[11]

Looking at a focused spinal assessment versus closed head injury may demand changes in Trendelenburg positions. All evaluations demand an effective proficiency not only in medicine but also in the technical aspects of mountain rescue.

As noted, this type of knowledge and technical skill acquisition goes beyond that typically learned in PA and NP programs or even medical school. Although many technical skills may be conveyed within specific rescue team training, students of medicine may find themselves gravitating toward wilderness/mountain medicine while enrolled in their traditional programs of study. In such environments, knowledge acquisition and training in mountain medicine may be initiated in student "interest groups" or more broadly in regional student wilderness medicine conferences. The WMS maintains resources connecting students with formal learning opportunities including student interest groups, student elective rotations, externships, and fellowships.[12] In addition to these resources, the WMS, working in collaboration with the University of Utah and AdventureMed, offers an AWLS certification course (https://adventuremed.com/).[13] This training highlights many of the foundational components of learning for those looking to practice mountain medicine. Beyond this tract, PAs, NPs, physicians, and medics may pursue more formal graduate-level education by obtaining a DiMM.[14] Offered by the military, the University of New Mexico, and the WMS, the DiMM is sanctioned by the International Commission of Alpine Rescue, which combines advanced practice care in consortium with the technical elements of mountain rescue.

Although the role of medical care in mountain rescue is often the focus of attention, there are other equally essential components. Administrative and organizational components of wilderness medicine are just as important. Within local Medical Rescue Association teams, medical personnel may find themselves used throughout the organizational structure. They may fill executive roles (ie, president), training roles, or even as a medical director. Some state boards of medicine have not yet considered PAs or NPs as medical directors, whereas in other states such roles are specifically permitted.[15] In North Carolina, both PAs and NPs may serve in the "assistant medical director" role. Although physicians may have the opportunity to take emergency medical services (EMS) fellowships, such training has not yet been broadly established for PAs and/or NPs. The concept of "Wilderness EMS" remains in its infancy of development, thereby leaving an area of opportunity for future PA and NP role growth. The American College of Emergency Physicians (ACEP) offers multiple policy statements considering the implementation of PAs and NPs but none speak to the role of the wilderness medicine provider.[16] The role of the PA/NP as an EMS medical director has only been generally described. Multiple PAs have attended the advanced medical director seminars of ACEP conferences.[17] These have included Wilderness EMS Medical Director courses to provide additional training for PAs and other providers aspiring to serve or collaborate in the medical direction of mountain rescue teams.

CASE

Although each rescue event is unique, an example can highlight roles and responsibilities. The following is a modified account of an actual technical mountain rescue.

The sheriff contacts the mountain rescue team via a phone app regarding a group of climbers who fell from the summit of the local mountain. Reportedly, one climber has fallen and is said to be "pretty banged up." Members of the team, who were previously enjoying a late Sunday afternoon, scramble to assemble gear and packs as they race to the mountain. All available teams meet at the base of the mountain within 2 hours. Updates are available via a rescue radio that also monitors traffic from the sheriff. The EMS phone app updates rescuers on avalanche conditions, patient demographics, and global positioning systems (GPS) coordinates for the last known position.

Once assembled at base, the sheriff notes that no helicopter resources will be available for the next 12 to 24 hours. A predeparture briefing and check lists are performed, ensuring all appropriate gear and resources have been collected. The team consists of two rescue leaders, three experienced field-team members, and two trainees. Snow is blowing sideways and the team base camp is approximately 5000 feet below the subjects. The sheriff contracts with a local snowcat to help shuttle the rescuers as high as possible; the rest of their journey will be on the icy slopes above. After exiting the snowcat, gear is carefully removed and distributed to the members—each carrying their load. Sticky "skins" are applied to their ski bottoms allowing the team to slide uphill on the snow. Radio contact is maintained with the base camp and the last known position of the subjects is reconfirmed. Navigating with compass and GPS, the team heads up hill as the twilight sunset embraces their journey.

Headlights of the rescuers can just barely be seen with binoculars from base as the blowing snow obscures the watchful eyes of the sheriff. As the team arrives to the plateau just below the summit, the entrance to the cave can be seen. This cave, which forms each climbing season, is a fumarole (see **Fig. 1**). The fumarole, containing toxic gasses (hydrogen sulfide, sulfur hydroxide, and carbon dioxide), has a very foul odor, which can be smelled from several hundred feet away. As the snow of the early summer melts, warm gasses from within the volcanic mountain erode from beneath the cave entrance. Eventually, the cave opens and presents an uninviting hazard to all climbers in the vicinity.

The rescue subject can be heard yelling from the dark abyss. Going into action, each member has pre-rehearsed tasks. The gas monitors come out to assess the fumarole conditions. Snow pickets are placed to create a robust array of rope anchors. Securely established, the rope rigging systems are assembled to bring the patient and rescuer back to safety.

One of the experienced medical volunteers prepares to enter the fumarole. His rigging is prepped for a hasty extraction, whereas the other experienced members will be designated as the edge attendant. The edge attendant performs predeparture safety checks and will be closely monitoring the gas monitors (see **Fig. 2**). If the gas monitors exceed the acceptable thresholds, the edge attendant must help coordinate immediate extraction with the gathered team above the fumarole. The rescuer descending into the fumarole is equipped with an APR mask and goggles. Equipment burdens, darkness, and the steam rising from the fumarole cave walls make the descent extremely dangerous.

As soon as the fallen climber is found, efforts are made in psychological first aid as he simultaneously tied into a harness, helmet, and APR mask. A quick evaluation of medical issues is done with concentration on the ABCs (airway, breathing, circulation) of emergency medicine. The airway is noted to be currently intact and the patient is responsive. An obvious angular deformity of the patient's left leg is noted, but further management and care will have to be performed after hasty removal from the fumarole environment.

Rope rescue at this position can mean being dragged up the crumbling wall of rock with the rescuer and the patient bound together. Adjustments are made at the top for a mechanical pulley device that tractors the climbers toward the top (**Fig. 4**).

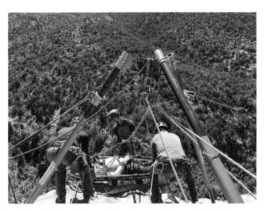

Fig. 4. Ropes used to extract fallen hiker. (*Courtesy of* Pearce Beissinger, used with permission; Fumarole, South Side of Mt Hood, Oregon.)

Every three feet of pull from the device gives one foot of rise to the rescue. The hazards of the toxic gas decrease as the patient and rescuer approach the surface of the cave. Incapacitated by pain, the patient is unable to facilitate any part of the vertical ascent and the rescuer must vector himself and the patient over the snowy lip of the cave using his legs. As is common, the snowy edge of the cave had been prepped with ice axes to facilitate this process.

At this point, the patient is reevaluated, splinted, packaged, and administered pain medication. Medical kits for mountain rescue are a medical committee decision and not decided without much deliberation. Efficacy, durability, weight, and efficiency must all be considered. A prefilled syringe of intramuscular ketamine is used to both decrease the pain and the memory of the rescue. A full body vacuum mattress is applied before further packaging into the rescue litter. Once clear of the fumarole, more rescue resources are now available. Attention is given not only to the orthopedic injury and gas exposure but also to the psychological stress injury from the event. Teams 2 and 3 have now arrived on scene with more supplies and personnel. The teams assemble a series of anchor stations where ropes operating in tandem allow rescuers to "leap frog" the litter down the mountain and to the awaiting snowcat, a few thousand feet below. The snowcat helps finish the journey back to the sheriff's base where care of the patient is transferred to the awaiting ambulance (**Fig. 5**).

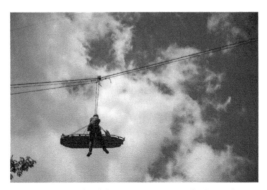

Fig. 5. Patient evacuation using "highlines" rigging technique (*Courtesy of* Pearce Beissinger, used with permission; Fumarole, South Side of Mt Hood, Oregon.)

SUMMARY

At the conclusion of each and every rescue, a debriefing is conducted by the team. Before heading home, an inventory of gear is checked and replaced. The Rescue leaders check on their members, assessing for signs of stress injury. Rescue teams have established a program for psychological first aid, not just for patients but for the rescuers that save them.[18] They make note of who might need follow-up. The cumulative stress of rescue work takes a toll on personnel as they return to their daily lives and family. Mitigating this burden has the goal of maintaining health, readiness, and the continued pursuit of team missions. Within hours of returning to base, a tired rescuer will push out a mission report to all team members reviewing the event, opportunities for improvement, and sometimes even an update from the patient's family. When rescuers leave the backcountry, the details of mountain rescue continue on the hearts and minds of each volunteer.

Rescue teams, like many in EMS, do not typically use the "safety first" philosophy, but instead "safety third." This concept acknowledges that rescue work is not safe. "Safety third" principals look to identify potential risks and injuries to mitigate their effects but allow the mission to be sustained.[19] Collectively using their unique skills, these "professional volunteers" selflessly serve the mountain community while passing on knowledge to future rescuers growing within their ranks.

CLINICS CARE POINTS

- Mountain rescue team members endure additional psychological stress injury that endures beyond a rescue and cumulatively affects their well-being.
- Mountain rescue team members are exposed to many environmental elements that threaten their health and safety.
- The rigors of mountain rescue demand that team members are well-versed in the technical and medical aspects of remote medical care.

DISCLOSURE

The views and written materials expressed in this publication do not necessarily represent the views of the United States Air Force, Department of Defense and/or the United States Government. Any mention of for profit training programs does not indicate support of the individual product or education program.

REFERENCES

1. Mountain Rescue Association, www.mra.org, Accessed 31 August, 2023.
2. Blancher M, Albasini F, Elsensohn F, et al. Management of multi-casualty incidents in mountain rescue: evidence-based guidelines of the international commission for mountain emergency medicine (ICAR MEDCOM). High Alt Med Biol 2018;19(2):131–40.
3. Hawkins S, editor. Wilderness. 1st ed. Philadelphia, PA: Wolters Kluwer, pub; 2017.
4. Sumann G, Moens D, Brink B, et al. Multiple trauma management in mountain environments - a scoping review: Evidence based guidelines of the International Commission for Mountain Emergency Medicine (ICAR MedCom). Intended for

physicians and other advanced life support personnel. Scand J Trauma Resusc Emerg Med 2020;28(1):117.

5. Volcanic air pollution and health, Center for Disease Control and Prevention, 2023, https://www.cdc.gov/air/volcanoes-air-pollution.htm, Accessed 31 August, 2023.

6. Luks AM, Auerbach PS, Freer L, et al. Wilderness Medical Society Practice Guidelines for the Prevention and Treatment of Acute Altitude Illness: 2019 Update. Wilderness Environ Med 2019;30(4).

7. Dzurisin D, Stauffer PH, Hendley JW II. Living with volcanic risk in the cascades. U.S. Geological Survey; 1997. revised 2008, Available at: https://pubs.usgs.gov/fs/1997/fs165-97/fs165-97.pdf. Accessed 12 September, 2023.

8. Occupational Safety and Health Administration, Fact Sheet Hydrogen Sulfide (H2S), https://www.osha.gov/sites/default/files/publications/hydrogen_sulfide_fact.pdf, Accessed 12 September, 2023.

9. Center for Disease Control and Prevention (CDC), National Institute of Occupational Safety and Health, Directory of Chemical Safety Resources, https://www.cdc.gov/niosh/topics/chemical.html, Accessed 12 September, 2023.

10. Ellerton J, Tomazin I, Brugger H, et al, For the International Commission for Mountain Emergency Medicine, International Commission for Mountain Emergency Medicine. Immobilization and splinting in mountain rescue Official Recommendations of the International Commission for Mountain Emergency Medicine, ICAR MEDCOM, Intended for Mountain Rescue First Responders, Physicians, and Rescue Organizations. High Alt Med Biol 2009 Winter;10(4):337–42.

11. Winterberger E, Jacomet H, Zafren K, et al. for the International Commission for Mountain Emergency Medicine; Terrestrial Rescue Commission of the International Commission for Alpine Rescue. The use of extrication devices in crevasse accidents: official statement of the International Commission for Mountain Emergency Medicine and the Terrestrial Rescue Commission of the International Commission for Alpine Rescue intended for physicians, paramedics, and mountain rescuers. Wilderness Environ Med 2008 Summer;19(2):108–10.

12. Wilderness Medical Society, students/residents, Austin, TX, https://wms.org/WMS/WMS/Learn/Student-Residents/Overview.aspx, Accessed 31 August, 2023.

13. AdventureMed, https://adventuremed.com/Accessed 12 September, 2023.

14. Wilderness Medical Society, Diploma in Mountain Medicine, https://wms.org/WMS/WMS/Get-Certified/DiMM/Overview.aspx, Accessed 31 August, 2023.

15. North Carolina College of Emergency Physicians Standards for the Selection and Performance of EMS Medical Director Requirements, https://www.ncems.org/pdf/SelectionandPerformanceofEMSMedicalDirectors.pdfAccessed 12 September, 2023.

16. American College of Emergency Physicians, Guidelines Regarding the Role of Physician Assistants and Nurse Practitioners in the Emergency Department, Updated June 23, 2023, https://www.acep.org/siteassets/new-pdfs/policy-statements/guidelines-reg-the-role-of-physician-assistants-and-nurse-practitioners-in-the-ed.pdf Accessed 12 September, 2023.

17. American College of Physicians, wilderness medicine section, https://www.acep.org/wilderness/resources, Accessed 31 August, 2023.

18. Responder Alliance, Buena Vista, CO, https://www.responderalliance.com/ Accessed 12 September, 2023.

19. Venter R. Safety First or Safety Third: Considering Practitioner Safety in EMS, 1/26/21. https://www.jems.com/commentary/safety-first-or-safety-third/, Accessed 12 September, 2023.

Medicine Under the Water
Dive Medicine

Kim Zuber, PA-C[a],*, Jane S. Davis, DNP[b]

KEYWORDS

- Diving injuries • DAN • Scuba • CDC yellow book • Veterans

KEY POINTS

- Diving injuries often occur in young, healthy participants.
- The vast majority of diving injuries occur during emergency ascent; diving deaths are usually related to running out of compressed gas.
- Divers Alert Network is the most complete worldwide source of diving mortality and morbidity data.

INTRODUCTION

There are more than 6 million self-contained underwater breathing apparatus (SCUBA) worldwide leading to more than 30 million dives per week.[1] The vast majority are young, healthy men (60%) aged younger than 30 years. Although this would lead one to think that dive medicine is not challenging, the Center for Disease Control and Prevention (CDC) notes that one in every 10 deaths of US travelers abroad is due to drowning.[2] Although several of these deaths may be related to swimming in rough, unknown waters or mixing alcohol and swimming, many are related to diving. For this reason, the CDC publishes a "yellow book" with a chapter highlighting *Scuba Diving: Decompression Illness & Other Dive-Related Injuries*.[3] In 2019, between 500,000 and 4 million Americans participated in recreational diving although the coronavirus disease 2019 pandemic severely curtailed this number in 2020 and 2021. Although all are required by law to complete at least the basic open water scuba diving course for diving certification, there are "shortcuts" at international resorts that allow a short intro course before a dive commences. Many other resorts will use professional divers to guide tourists through a dive experience.[4]

Diving History

Archaeologists have found evidence of humans gathering sponges, food, pearls, and even corals as far back as 4500 to 3200 BC.[5] Diving was used for military purposes during the Trojan Wars in 1194 BC. By the early third century BC, Aristotle and Alexander the Great were writing of a "*diving bell*" allowing divers to breathe below the water

[a] American Academy of Nephrology PAs, Melbourne, FL, USA; [b] Nephrology, University of Alabama at Birmingham, Birmingham, AL, USA
* Corresponding author.
E-mail address: zuberkim@yahoo.com

Physician Assist Clin 9 (2024) 311–319
https://doi.org/10.1016/j.cpha.2023.08.007
2405-7991/24/© 2023 Elsevier Inc. All rights reserved.

surface. The first reports of dive medical issues occurred around this time with reports of tympanic membrane pain due to water pressure.[5]

Commercial diving came into use in the second century BC with the development of a snorkel-type device.[5] A hood snorkel was developed by Leonardo Da Vinci in the fifteenth century with small modifications made during the next 200 years. The SCUBA suit, introduced in 1825, lead to the introduction of the term "frog-men" into the general lexicon.[5,6] SCUBA diving as we know it came into existence in the twentieth century with the invention of compressed air in cylinder tanks and a regulator.[5] SCUBA and the military have been intertwined for many years. Divers in World War II were an essential part of the war effort. They planted explosives, neutralized depth charges, and cleared beaches for the Navy Seals.[6]

Medical Issues

Under the water, objects seem 25% larger, sound travels 4 times faster and heat is conducted 25% faster than on land.[7] The color spectrum will disappear into complete darkness as one descends with red being the last color lost. As one gets deeper underwater, water gets colder with column thermoclines delineated. Water pressure increases 1 atm every 33 feet of depth or twice as much as it would be if one was on land. Thus, diving deaths and accidents are often caused by significantly different issues than those on land (**Table 1**). Diver Alert Network (DAN) collects and publishes morbidity and mortality statistics. It also offers emergency medical advice if a diver or diving company gets into trouble.

Aristotle was the first to describe issues with ears and diving but he would not be the last.[3,5] The CDC notes that barotrauma is the most common injury in divers. If one does not equalize pressures within the middle ear as one descends, the middle ear tissues will swell and force equalization (IE: Valsalva maneuver) can actually cause tympanic rupture. However, there are usually preceding symptoms before trauma that can warn the diver to ascend:[3]

Table 1
Dive Complications reported to DAN 2014–2018[8]

Complication	2014–2017 (Mean)	2018 (Count)
Barotrauma	1008	1053
Decompression sickness	606	624
Marine envenomation	234	202
Immersion pulmonary edema (IPE)	46	47
Arterial gas embolism (AGE)	40	41
Fatality	41	18
Nonfatal drowning	23	17
Gas contamination	22	18
Fin foot (reactive hyperemia)	18	13
Motion sickness	14	24
Mask squeeze	15	5
Loss of consciousness	11	5
Cardiac arrhythmia	7	0
Nitrogen narcosis	3	2

Abbreviation: DAN, Diver Alert Network.
Adapted from Tillmans F. DAN Annual Diving Report 2020 Edition-A report on 2018 diving fatalities, injuries and incidents. Durham, NC: Divers Alert Network, 2020, pp22, used with permission.

- Pain
- Tinnitus (ringing in the ears)
- Vertigo (dizziness or sensation of spinning)
- Sensation of fullness
- Sense of "water" in the ear (serous fluid/blood accumulation in the middle ear)
- Decreased hearing[3]

Although the invention of self-contained breathing systems was an advance by allowing tanks of gas to be carried to wherever the diver wished to go, the use of compressed gas has also increased lung trauma. Lung trauma usually occurs if ascending is too fast and "*gas bubbles*" are trapped. If gas bubbles form, they can move into 3 different spaces:[3]

- Pleural space
- Pulmonary vasculature
- Mediastinum

The most dangerous of these is the movement of gas bubbles into the pleural space and/or into pulmonary vasculature. This can cause a pneumothorax and the need for a chest tube. If the gas bubbles move into the pulmonary vasculature, they can enter the left side of the heart and cause an arterial gas embolism (AGE). AGE requires hyperbaric treatment and is considered a dive emergency. Subcutaneous emphysema ("bubbles" in the mediastinum) can cause pain, temporary voice changes, and that uncomfortable feeling of fullness in the chest.

The first person to describe decompression illness was Robert Boyle in 1670.[5] Boyle theorized that due to underwater pressure, air bubbles push into the bloodstream and obstruct blood flow. Andrew Smith, an ear, nose and throat (ENT) surgeon, described more than 100 cases of decompression sickness during the Brooklyn Bridge project in the nineteenth century. Because the most prevalent symptoms are joint pain and bent posture, decompression sickness became known as "*doing the bends*."[5] In 1915, the United States Navy introduced a diving table, recommending stops during ascending and mandating maximum operating depth on compressed atmospheric air and pure oxygen.[5] We now know that decompression illness actually describes 2 different entities: vascular injury such as AGE and decompression sickness. Clinically both present similarly but there are differences (**Table 2**). Treatment, after identification, includes immediate transfer to a facility with a hyperbaric chamber.

AGE and decompression sickness are not the only pulmonary issues that can develop. Nitrogen narcosis can be life threatening. It occurs at deeper depths although it clears on ascent, which differentiates it from AGE. However, the narcosis can cause divers to remove their mask or breathing apparatus and death occurs by drowning. Another serious pulmonary issue is immersion or induced pulmonary edema (IPE) which can cause excess fluid to be pushed into the lungs. This can present on descent or at depth as chest pain, dyspnea, wheezing, and productive cough with frothy sputum.[3] Divers are warned that risks increase with age, left ventricular hypertrophy, and overhydration. A predive physical will consider all medical conditions with increased concentration on the pulmonary system.

Although the issues above are life threatening, other less fatal risks are also present:[3]

- Seizures caused by dropping partial pressures of oxygen in the bloodstream
- Toxic marine life
- Fatal injuries from marine life (sharks, barbs, bacterial contamination, and so forth)[9]

Table 2
Clinical findings of decompression illness

Arterial Gas Embolism	Decompression Sickness
Chest pain or bloody sputum	Coughing spasms or shortness of breath
Loss of consciousness	Collapse of unconsciousness
Personality change, difficulty thinking, or confusion	Personality change
Muscular weakness	Weakness
Numbness or paresthesia	Numbness or Tingling
Dizziness	Dizziness
Paralysis	Paralysis
Ataxia	Staggering, loss of coordination, or tremors
Blurred vision	Mottling or marbling of skin
Convulsions	Loss of bowel or bladder function
	Itching
	Joint aches or pain
	Unusual fatigue

Adapted from Nord AD, Raczniak AG, Chimiak J. Travelers' Health, chap 3: Scuba Diving: Decompression Illness & Other Dive-Related Injuries, chart 3.4. https://wwwnc.cdc.gov/travel/yellowbook/2018/the-pre-travel-consultation/scuba-diving, Accessed 26Jul2022.

Dive and fly trips often mean that a diver will get into a pressurized plane after diving. Although there are no strict rules for diving after flying, for the reverse (flying after diving), there are specific directions. One needs to wait at least 12 hours after a single no-compression dive, 48 hours after multiple days of diving and 24 to 48 hours after any compression dive.[10]

Medical Clearance

In 1977, the Undersea and Hyperbaric Society (UHMS) of the National Oceanic and Atmospheric Administration (NOAA) cooperated with the US Navy to design a standardized training course for physicians who wanted to specialize in dive medicine. NOAA continues to develop and update Diving Medical Standards and Procedures. As of 2010, the evaluation of the prospective diver can be done by an MD, DO, PA, or NP certified by NOAA.[11] Besides a history and physical, laboratory and further testing are mandated depending on diver's age (**Table 3**). Recertification for diving requires testing to be repeated at specific intervals, again dependent on age.

As more patients with diabetes are encouraged to increase exercise, some have turned to diving. DAN has specific protocols for patients with diabetes although these have not been updated since 2005.[12] They do require patients to be stable and on insulin for more than 1 year or oral medications more than 3 months before attempting to dive. Blood sugar checks are mandated at specific intervals.

Medical Care

DAN is a nonprofit organization that has collected data and monitored diving since 1980.[13] As diving is a worldwide sport with many levels of participation, often injuries or causes of morbidity and mortality are not reported. DAN is the most complete database available. In late 2022, the most recent data published (**Table 4**), diving-related fatalities were mainly caused by gas issues:[8,14]

Table 3
Minimum physical examination for diving clearance (2010)

Initial Physical (all Ages)	Periodic Physical (all Ages)
Medical history and physical examination	Medical history and physical examination
Complete blood count (CBC)	CBC
Urinalysis (micro if indicated)	Urinalysis (micro if indicated)
Vision (corrected/uncorrected)	Vision (Corrected/uncorrected)
Height and weight	Height and weight
Spirometry	Spirometry (if a smoker)
Chest x-ray within 24 months	
Audiometry	
Additional tests 40 y and older	*Additional tests 40 y and older*
12-lead electrocardiogram (EKG)	12-lead EKG
Fasting blood lipid panel	Fasting blood lipid panel
Hemoglobin A1C	Hemoglobin A1C

Adapted from National Association of Oceanic and Atmospheric Administration (NOAA) Diving Medical Standards and Procedures Manual, https://www.omao.noaa.gov/learn/headquarters/office-health-services/diving-medicine, The NOAA Diving Program, 2010, Accessed 27Jul2022.

For patients who survive the ascent but show signs of *"the bends"* caused by either AGE or decompression sickness, hyperbaric oxygen (HBO) therapy is the mainstay of treatment. Most of the treatment protocols have been developed by the UHMS.[15,16] The UHMS has more than 2000 physician, scientist, associate, and nurse members. They are a source of peer-reviewed articles as well as symposia, courses, and workshops along with an annual meeting. While headquartered in Florida, they have international members from more than 30 countries.

HBO treatment uses pressured oxygen to shrink the size of the systemic gas bubbles found in decompression injury thus allowing for elimination of the dissolved gases.[14] Hard cylinder chambers can be single chambers or larger room-type chambers. Chambers are found on ships that transport divers, especially in the military, and in many hospital systems, especially those close to the coasts. During the years, the UHMS has developed and refined HBO protocols for divers while also developing many other medical uses for HBO, mainly in the area of wound infections.[16]

Table 4
Causes of diving deaths 2019 and 2020

Causes of Diving Deaths in 2019	Causes of Diving Deaths in 2020
Running out of breathing gas (41%)	Unknown (55%)
Entrapment (21%)	Natural disease (9%)
Equipment problems (15%)	Equipment problems (9%)
Rough water (10%)	Rapid ascent (8%)
Trauma (6%)	Arrhythmia due to methamphetamine (4%)
Buoyancy (4%)	Buoyancy (2%)
Inappropriate gas (3%)	Insufficient gas (6%)

Abbreviation: DAN, Diver Alert Network.
Adapted from DAN.[8,14]

Diving and Traditional Complementary Medicine

Traditional complementary medicine (TCM) has ventured into dive medicine but mostly at the periphery. One notable book, *Diving Medical Acupuncture: Treatment and Prevention of Diving Medical Problems*, highlighted treatment and prevention of ear disorders for divers.[17] This book is valuable for TCM practitioners, both divers and nondivers. Since approximately 70% of diving related illnesses involve ENT, TCM is an alternative to the usual treatments and procedures offered by ENT practitioners. Some mild ENT deformities or illnesses can be troublesome in diving. Issues include the following:

- Common cold
- Rhinosinusitis
- Allergic rhinitis
- Mucous membranes hyperactivity
- Deviated septum
- Cyst
- Tumor
- Enlarged lingual/pharyngeal tonsils
- Polyps
- Turbinate hypertrophy
- Excess cerumen
- Sinus infections

Although acupuncture and herbal medicine cannot change congenital structural defects, TCM can focus on particular ENT issues.[18] An example is the "*Shang Han Lun*," which uses 6 stages to treat the common cold or influenza. This is accomplished by differentiating wind-cold and wind-heat from others. By expelling wind, strengthening *Wei qi* and addressing the underlying 6 evils, divers can opt to receive a natural alternative treatment rather than medication, which may wear off during the dive.[18] Issues with seasickness, vertigo, and/or upset stomachs may be treated with TCM highlighting the *liver qi stagnation.* This is treated with acupuncture and herbs with the TCM practitioner deciding on the appropriate herbal formula, the timing, the frequency of dosing. Although severe diving emergencies, decompression sickness, and/or AGE are out of the scope of TCM and need HBO therapy, TCM modalities can assist the diver both after the incident and before the next dive.[18]

The largest group of divers who benefit from acupuncture is those with chronic pain conditions, arthritis, muscular pain, and/or autoimmune-related pain.[18] Although some of these conditions may keep divers from being certified by a dive physical, many others can be managed without medication by the TCM practitioner. For many dive enthusiasts, diving allows them to see a completely different world; acupuncture treatment may help with chronic pain opening the sport to many more people.

TCM modalities such as acupuncture and herbal medicine play an essential role in controlling and preventing inflammation.[19] Recognizing this, TCM has been implemented into ENT clinics in Australia with good results. However, there is a difference in treatment regimens. For patients who are symptomatic on both land and sea and have visible signs of inflammation, treatments are often longer than for those who are only symptomatic in the water.[19]

Diving and Veterans

In 2019, the CDC introduced a Comprehensive Suicide Prevention Program with special attention to populations at disproportionate risk for suicide.[20] This included veterans. Community-based programs were to highlight *"connectiveness with peer norm programs and community engagement."* Multiple nonprofit, community-based dive programs for veterans have been active for several years and fit into the CDC suicide prevention programs.[21–23] However, although the programs state that they do help with suicide prevention, less formal research has been done with these programs. Yet participants described the feeling of being in a peer group as therapeutic. The groups showed excellent camaraderie. Amputees and those with physical disabilities appreciated the ability to not be limited by prosthetics.

To address this lack of controlled data collection, a formalized research study was conducted in the United Kingdom specific to veterans who participated in scuba diving programs.[24] Using the General Health Questionnaire (GHQ-28) predive and postdive sessions, the veterans showed a statistically significant 14.3-point increase in the GHQ-28 scores. Scuba diving offered significant therapeutic benefits and these were more prominent in the ex-military amputee population. Scuba, as a therapy, was found to have a positive outcome in the following:

- The need for complete focus
- The feeling of weightlessness underwater; this was most evident in the amputee population
- Assisted in the relief of chronic pain
- Assisted in the lessening of depression symptoms

DIVE MEDICINE

Diving has a long eventful history dating back to the prehistoric period. What began from necessity and curiosity still continuously drives human beings into the depths of the ocean. Whether the purpose is to defend a nation, mount an invasion or to meet the creatures of the deep from myths and stories, diving is more and more mainstream. With technology advancement and more affordable prices, there are more divers resulting in more diving-related medical issues. Diving originated in areas of the world that use Eastern medicine and although studies are not published in typical Western medicine journals, there is a wealth of knowledge and training in TCM available. TCM is effective in treating and preventing respiratory and ENT conditions both on land and in water.[19] TCM can be a valuable, cost-effective adjunct for traditional dive remedies. As always, more research is needed.

CLINICS CARE POINTS

- Because of the difference between land and water, medical issues in water are commonly barotrauma, decompression sickness and marine envenomation; these are less likely in land medicine.
- Arterial gas embolism vs decompression sickness is difficult to distinguish clinically. However, the treatment is the same: a hyperbaric chamber.
- The National Oceanic and Atmospheric Administration (NOAA) has developed certification for a dive medical clearance that can be done by an MD, DO, PA or NP.

ACKNOWLEDGMENTS

A very special thank you to Dr Kenneth Huynh A. P, D.O.M, D.A.C.M of the Tampa Bay Spearfishing Club for his expert assistance.

DISCLOSURE

None.

REFERENCES

1. Fulbrook P. Deep Dive Scuba.com, Diving Statistics2022, http://divedeepscuba.com/scuba-diving-statistics-2022/, Accessed 27 July, 2022.
2. Center for Disease and Control and Prevention, Swimming and Diving Safety, https://wwwnc.cdc.gov/travel/page/safe-swimming-diving, CDC, Atlanta GA, Accessed 26 July, 2022.
3. Nord AD, Raczniak AG, Chimiak J. Travelers' Health, chap 3: Scuba Diving: Decompression Illness & Other Dive-Related Injuries, https://wwwnc.cdc.gov/travel/yellowbook/2018/the-pre-travel-consultation/scuba-diving, Accessed 26 July, 2022.
4. Professional association of dive instructors (PADI), https://www.padi.com/, Accessed 26 July, 2022.
5. Acott C. A brief history of diving and decompression illness. https://www.semanticscholar.org/paper/A-brief-history-of-diving-and-decompression-Acott/f13e5a899cec8f6dcddf97fd24c72ffd710cf183, 1999, Psychol, Corpus ID: 56703033
6. Modern Marvel Scuba diving history by modern marvels, History Channel, https://www.history.com/shows/modern-marvels/season-5/episode-11, Accessed 21 October, 2017
7. Scuba Diving International (SDI). Open water scuba diver, https://www.tdisdi.com/, Accessed 24 January, 2019.
8. Tillmans F. DAN Annual Diving Report 2020 Edition-A report on 2018 diving fatalities, injuries and incidents. Durham, NC: Divers Alert Network; 2020. p. pp22.
9. Acott CJ. Sea-snake envenomation. Med J Aust 1986;144(8):448.
10. Vann RD. Guidelines for flying after diving, Proceedings Summary DAN Flying After Diving Workshop, https://dan.org/health-medicine/health-resource/health-safety-guidelines/guidelines-for-flying-after-diving/, Accessed 26 August, 2022.
11. National Association of Oceanic and Atmospheric Administration (NOAA). Diving medical Standards and procedures Manual. The NOAA Diving Program; 2010. https://www.omao.noaa.gov/learn/headquarters/office-health-services/diving-medicine. Accessed 27 July, 2022.
12. Diabetes and recreational diving: guidelines for the future. In: Pollock NW, Uguccioni DM, Dear GdeL, editors. Proceedings of the UHMS/DAN 2005 June 19 workshop. Durham, NC: Divers Alert Network; 2005.
13. Divers Alert Network, Duke University, https://dan.org/, Accessed 8 July, 2023.
14. Divers Alert Network, Dive Accident Insurance, https://www.diversalertnetwork.org/insurance/dive/, Accessed 26 February, 2019.
15. Undersea and Hyperbaric Medical Society, https://www.uhms.org/, Accessed 27 July, 2022.
16. U.S. Navy Diving Manual, Volume 5: Diving Medicine and Recompression Chamber Operations, 2008, http://www.usu.edu/scuba/navy_manual6.pdf, Accessed 29 July, 2022.
17. Vermeulen J. Diving medical acupuncture: treatment and prevention of diving medical Problems with a focus on ENT disorders. 1st edition. Singing Dragon Publications; 2018.
18. Deadman P, Al-Khafaji M, Baker K. A Manual of Acupuncture, J Chin Med, 2nd edition 1998, digital version https://amanualofacupuncture.com/digital-member

ship/, Crushing Malloy, Inc., Ann Arbor, Michigan, USA, 2000. ISBN-13: 978-0951054659, ISBN-10: 0951054651, Accessed 5 July, 2022.

19. Nabil WN, Zhou W, Shergis JL, et al. Management of respiratory disorders in a Chinese medicine teaching clinic in Australia: review of clinical records. Chin Med 2015;10:31.

20. Jones C. CDC testimony on reducing Military and veteran suicide. Washington DC: Acting Director of National Center for Injury Prevention and Control; 2022. https://www.cdc.gov/washington/testimony/2022/t20220615.htm. Accessed 7 July, 2023.

21. Dive Therapy for Veterans, https://www.vetdivetherapy.com/, Accessed 7 July, 2023.

22. Dive4Vets Foundation, https://dive4vets.org/about/, Accessed 7 July, 2023.

23. WAVES Project, https://www.wavesproject.org/, Accessed 7 July, 2023.

24. Morgan A, Sinclair H, Tan A, et al. Can scuba diving offer therapeutic benefit to military veterans experiencing physical and psychological injuries as a result of combat? A service evaluation of Deptherapy UK. Disabil Rehabil 2019;41(23): 2832–40.

Interdisciplinary Wilderness Medicine Education

Eric Olsen, PA-C[a], Stephanie Lareau, MD[a,b],*

KEYWORDS

- Wilderness medicine education • Interdisciplinary medical education • MedWAR
- Wilderness medicine electives

KEY POINTS

- Care for patients in austere environments often involves interdisciplinary teams.
- Opportunities for interdisciplinary training exist through electives, specialty courses, competitions, and fellowships.
- Interdisciplinary training, especially in wilderness medicine, has the potential to improve both care in the field and with the hospital and in the clinic.
- Care in wilderness environments often involves interdisciplinary teams of medical providers. Within medical education opportunities are often siloed; this is true to some extent within wilderness medicine. There are opportunities including commercially available courses, MedWAR competitions, Wilderness Medical Society fellowships, and wilderness medicine electives that foster interdisciplinary learning.
- Interdisciplinary skills learning in wilderness medicine can be applied throughout health care environments.

INTRODUCTION

The complexities of patient care in austere environments drive the need for effective interdisciplinary collaboration.[1] With a team of multiple professions and different specialties within those professions, it is important that everyone involved can work together to achieve a common goal. Training for this level of collaboration starts in each respective discipline's professional schooling. There are different modalities for interdisciplinary education. One option is for medical students, physician assistant (PA) students, nursing students, and/or paramedic students to participate in group classes or problem-based situations. This is beneficial as it allows all participants to have a common shared knowledge and shared experiences to draw from in the future. Another option is to have the students participate in preceptorship with an experienced and knowledgeable practitioner in one of the other disciples. This allows the

a Department of Emergency Medicine, Carilion Clinic 1906 Belleview Avenue, Roanoke, VA 24014, USA; b Virginia Tech Carilion School of Medicine, 2 Riverside Circle, Roanoke, VA 24016, USA
* Corresponding author. 1906 Belleview Avenue, Roanoke VA 24014.
E-mail address: salareau@carilionclinic.org

Physician Assist Clin 9 (2024) 321–325
https://doi.org/10.1016/j.cpha.2023.08.010
2405-7991/24/© 2023 Elsevier Inc. All rights reserved.

physicianassistant.theclinics.com

student to appreciate contributions made by other team members. The student will also experience the inner workings of those other professions involved in patient care. Ideally, this will lead to patience, empathy, and increased trust amongst teammates.

Interdisciplinary learning helps to foster an attitude of mutual respect and eagerness for collaboration. Wilderness medicine (WM) incidents often have very limited resources. This makes understanding and effective communication with colleagues critical to success. There is an increased likelihood of any given situation involving higher levels of stress involved due to the strenuous nature of care in austere environments. The rescuers themselves are often exposed to the same environmental extremes that contributed to creating an emergency situation. Heat or cold exposure, dehydration, and physical exertion can increase stress making it even more important for each member of a team to know the capabilities of others ahead of time. The interdisciplinary learning environment instills a greater appreciation for what their colleagues from other departments can contribute.

Initial health care training in general and specifically in WM often occurs in a more siloed approach, where paramedic students work with other paramedic students and medical students work with other medical students. Student interest groups in WM are typically based at medical or PA schools and only include students in that program. Interest groups are an affordable and effective way to introduce students to WM, as they work with student schedules.[2]

In some residency programs, physicians do have the opportunity to learn WM topics during emergency training. Within an emergency medicine residency there is no official curriculum established for WM; however, topics such as hyperbaric medicine are part of the core curriculum. Studies show 44% of emergency medicine programs do offer an option for WM electives.[3] Additionally, residents from all programs can take advantage of rotations away from their institution, including Wilderness Medicine Society Resident Electives or clinical opportunities at ski clinics.

Other electives have focused more specifically on interprofessional education. A 2 week elective at Johns Hopkins paired medical students with non-physician preceptors, including nurses, pharmacists, and physical therapists from different departments within the health care team. During the elective students rotated with experienced preceptors in nursing, social work, rehabilitation therapy, pharmacy, hospital administration and infection control, home care, and palliative care. The study demonstrated that the experience empowered students to provide coordinated care and collaborate more effectively.[4] Students who participate in interprofessional extracurricular activities, especially patient based ones such as global health trips, were shown to have better attitudes toward interprofessional education.[5]

In a study of simulated scenarios at a rural WM conference, the wilderness environment was also identified as a key factor in facilitating sharing. Sharing was the core concept that allowed participants to develop strategies for developing common goals, partaking in leadership and developing mutual respect and understanding.[6]

Beyond the initial individual trainings and residency programs, another opportunity for interprofessional education is the pursuit of *Fellow of the Academy of Wilderness Medicine (FAWM)*. FAWM is awarded by the Wilderness Medical Society and is open to all medical providers who have graduated from one of the specified health care professions and completed 1 year of practice in their discipline. The core group of requirements includes earning credits from attending didactic lectures, obtaining experiences and performing service within WM. Although this is an individual pursuit, to satisfy the requirements, the candidates will have to complete their course work alongside people of all backgrounds. The knowledge that everyone who has completed a FAWM has been trained to the same standard, regardless of professional title, can help establish trust among WM practitioners.

WM fellowships also exist as 1 or 2 year long graduate medical education programs for physicians in emergency medicine, family medicine, and internal medicine. As of April 2023, there were 22 WM fellowships. The curriculum in WM fellowships covers altitude illness, environmental exposures, trauma, expeditions, dive medicine and drowning, envenomation, search and rescue, survival, lightning strikes, avalanche, and wilderness toxicology.[3]

There are 2 WM fellowships offered within the United States for PAs and nurse practitioners (NPs), Virginia Tech Carilion (WM) Fellowship and the Medical College of Georgia WM Fellowship. They adhere to a similar curriculum as the physician fellowships and their PA/NP fellows have the option to complete similar courses and field experiences. These programs foster an environment for collaborative learning. Physicians, PAs, and NPs participate together in didactics, expedition trips, certification courses, and outreach programs. They learn to rely on one another and to value each other's strengths. Fellows often go on to remain involved in the program, training future aspirants.

Outside of traditional academics, there are commercially available WM courses. These courses are tailored to the scope of practice of the individual. Courses such as *Wilderness First Responder* and *Wilderness First Aid* are geared to the lay person. There are also courses such as *Wilderness Life Support–Medical Providers* and *Wilderness Upgrade for Medical Providers* that are designed for health care professionals including emergency medical technicians (EMTs), registered nurses (RNs), PAs, NPs, and physicians. These courses incorporate interdisciplinary learning into the wilderness medical arena. With medical professionals from different backgrounds learning and honing their skills together, it more closely approximates the real-world situation. The Diploma in Mountain Medicine is governed by the Union Internationale des Association d'Alpinisme (UIAA) and is open to health care professionals including physicians, RNs, NPs, PAs, paramedics, and advanced EMTs. It is a 120 hour course to prepare medical professionals to provide medical care in mountain environments. It includes technical skills: rope rescue in a vertical environment, crevasse rescue, and helicopter operations. This course is offered in 25 locations including the United States, Europe, Nepal, and Japan.

An opportunity to incorporate a diverse group of health care practitioners occurs with the Medical Wilderness Adventure Races, MedWAR (https://www.medwar.org/). These events are set in beautiful locations across the country and are open to teams of 3 to 4 participants from a variety of backgrounds. Participants typically register as a team. Participants can be practicing medical providers, students or wilderness enthusiast without formal training. Teams are required to use orienteering to make their way between checkpoints, traveling by hiking, biking, or paddling. Once they arrive at the checkpoints, the participants are tested on either general WM knowledge or presented with a hands-on scenario where they will be rendering aid to a victim.[7] These events are a great opportunity for health care providers to complement each other's strengths and weaknesses as they compete toward a common goal.

As interprofessionalism is important in WM delivery, faculty at Virginia Tech Carilion School of Medicine and Radford University Carilion designed an elective to bring together medical students, PA students, and paramedic students. This elective is unique in that it has medical students, PA students, and paramedic students complete the elective together. It is designed as a 2 week experience for fourth year medical students, second year PA students, and final year paramedic students. During the first day of the elective, students complete team building activities together including a navigation challenge and they learn the basics of patient assessment in a wilderness environment using the Massive Hemorrhage, Airway, Respirations/Breathing, Circulation, Hypothermia/Hyperthermia/Hike/Helicopter (MARCH) algorithm. MARCH is accepted by the American College of Surgeons in the Advanced Trauma Life Support curriculum as well as the Committee on Tactical Combat Casualty Care for assessing an injured person.

During the WM elective, students complete the *Wilderness Life Support for Medical Provider's* course, the *American Canoe Association Level 3 River Safety Course*, participate in a caving trip, learn basic rope rescue skills, and have opportunities to work alongside WM faculty providing race support. Course instructors include physicians, PAs, NPs, and paramedics who are all active locally in WM. It is important for learners to have role models within their specific profession. Our goal is to involve those in WM leadership roles so students can fully understand their potential involvement.

Students from each discipline bring unique skills to scenarios. A general impression is that the medical and PA students have more basic science knowledge, whereas the paramedic students bring more practical skills in patient assessment and transport in the austere environment. Paramedic students generally have more hands-on experience with patient care, assessment, splinting, patient packaging, and patient transport. Medical and PA students typically have a deeper understanding of the pathophysiology of conditions discussed and the in-hospital care. Our real-world experience has shown us that when you are on scene in an austere environment all these things are important. Students will learn from each other while complimenting the others skill set.

The goal of our elective and all the programs described above are to break out of our individual silos of learning and learn from each other. By creating interdisciplinary opportunities within WM, we hope that these experiences will not only translate into improved care for patients in wilderness environments, but teamwork and collaboration skills will also translate back to the hospital environment as well. The obstacles and challenges faced when working in the field can build teamwork and resilience.

CLINICS CARE POINTS

- In austere environments, interdisiplinary teams are common.
- Interdisiplinary training has potential to improve patient care in austere environments.
- Opportunities exist for PAs to gain interdisiplinary training through courses and formal fellowships.

DISCLOSURE

The authors have nothing to disclose.

REFERENCES

1. Russell KW, Weber DC, Scheele BM, et al. Search and Rescue in the Intermountain West States. Wilderness Environ Med 2013;24(4):429–33.
2. Fielding CM. Introducing Medical Students to Wilderness Medicine. Wilderness Environ Med 2011;22(1):91–3.

3. Holstrom-Mercader M, Kass D, Corsetti M, et al. Wilderness Medicine Curricula in United States EMS Fellowship, Emergency Medicine Residency, and Wilderness Medicine Programs. Prehosp Disaster Med 2022;37(6):800–5.
4. Pathak S, Holzmueller CG, Haller KB, et al. A Mile in Their Shoes: Interdisciplinary Education at the Johns Hopkins University School of Medicine. Am J Med Qual 2010;25(6):462–7.
5. Wong RL, Fahs DB, Talwalkar JS, et al. A longitudinal study of health professional students' attitudes towards interprofessional education at an American university. J Interprof Care 2016;30(2):191–200.
6. Smith HA, Reade M, Maar M, et al. Developing a grounded theory for interprofessional collaboration acquisition using facilitator and actor perspectives in simulated wilderness medical emergencies. Rural Rem Health 2017;17(1):1–7. Available at: https://search.informit.org/doi/10.3316/informit.151132048501712.
7. Ledrick DJ. The Medical Wilderness Adventure Race (MedWAR): a 2-year perspective on a unique learning experience. Wilderness Environ Med 2003; 14(4):273–6.

Moving?

Make sure your subscription moves with you!

To notify us of your new address, find your **Clinics Account Number** (located on your mailing label above your name), and contact customer service at:

Email: journalscustomerservice-usa@elsevier.com

800-654-2452 (subscribers in the U.S. & Canada)
314-447-8871 (subscribers outside of the U.S. & Canada)

Fax number: 314-447-8029

Elsevier Health Sciences Division
Subscription Customer Service
3251 Riverport Lane
Maryland Heights, MO 63043

*To ensure uninterrupted delivery of your subscription, please notify us at least 4 weeks in advance of move.

ELSEVIER

Printed and bound by CPI Group (UK) Ltd, Croydon, CR0 4YY

03/10/2024

01040847-0015